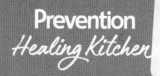

Healthy Smoothies

100+ Delicious Recipes for Optimal Wellness

HEARST
HOME

Prevention
Healing Kitchen

Contents

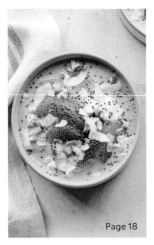

Page 18

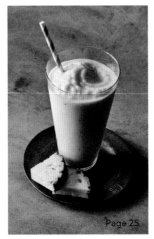

Page 25

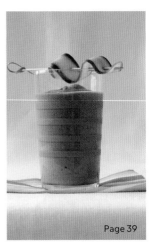

Page 39

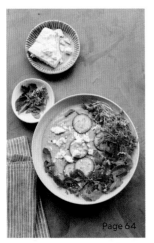

Page 64

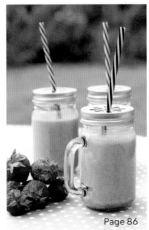

Page 86

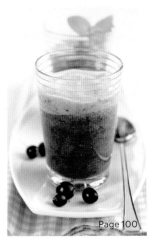

Page 100

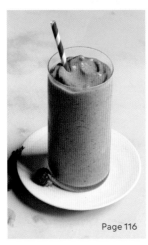

Page 116

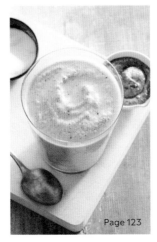

Page 123

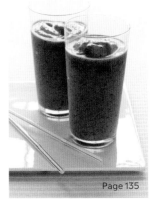

Page 135

Foreword

When I talk to clients and friends about what keeps them from eating healthier, their reasons often come down to time. There are just too few hours in the day to meet all of their commitments and also cook healthy meals. It's true that making your own nutrient-packed meals can take time each week that many of us just can't spare. But a simple solution is probably already in your kitchen: a blender. If you have this versatile appliance, you can be a smoothie master! Delicious, nutritious meals-to-go can be made in just minutes.

A smoothie can be an energizing, on-the-go breakfast, a between-meal pick-me-up, or even part of your pre-bedtime ritual to help you relax. Endlessly adaptable, smoothies can help keep you nourished and balanced, no matter what the world throws your way.

Since I know you're looking to optimize your health with the food you put in your body, we've categorized the smoothies into chapters for specific health concerns, from gut health to athletic performance. Whether you're a busy working mom or a time-strapped student, this book will help you find smoothie solutions that fit your life. I'll drink to that!

—Frances Largeman-Roth, RDN
Nutritionist, mom, and wellness expert

Tools and Techniques

Get set to blend your healthiest, most flavorful smoothies with a few helpful kitchen tools, tips, and ingredient picks.

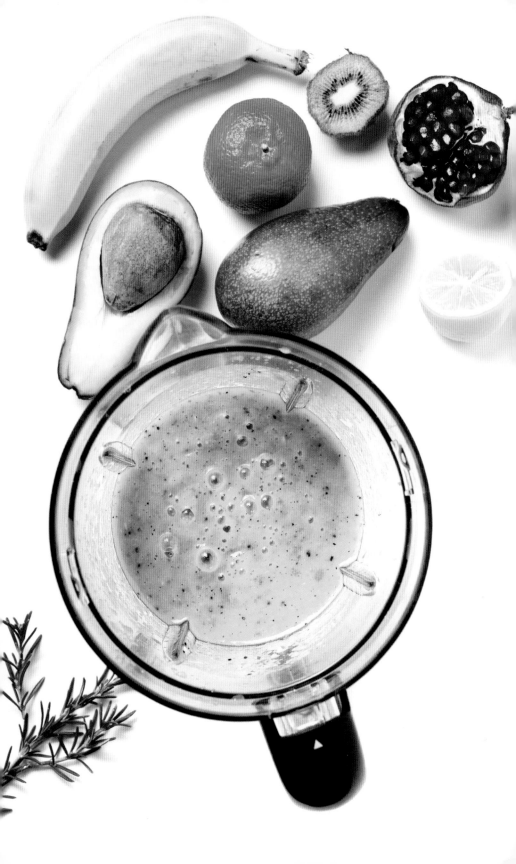

KITCHEN ESSENTIALS

If you already have a blender on hand, you're ready to go. If you're still in the market for one, read ahead to pick the best style for your needs.

A traditional blender features a heavy metal base topped by a plastic or glass blending container. The latest models are sturdy and high-powered and have multiple settings that make it easy to achieve consistently blended smoothies. Though you usually are advised not to clean the container in the dishwasher, it can often be washed quickly by filling it with water, adding a few drops of dish detergent, and giving it a spin on the base.

Try to wash it soon after blending to avoid a caked-on mess!

If you want to be able to prep your smoothies in advance, it's nice to have a "personal" blender. This style of appliance has a cup that attaches directly to the base. You can use the cup to prepare your ingredients the night before, so all you need to do is roll out of bed, blend, and go! Some blenders are sold with both a traditional container and a to-go cup, which provides great versatility.

While a blender is all you need to combine your ingredients, some additional accessories will help you prep.

1. CHEF'S KNIFE:
This is crucial for smoothie prep, from cutting melons in half and chopping nuts to dicing carrots.

2. CITRUS ZESTER:
This type of grater removes only the colorful outer peel from citrus fruits. It can also be used to grate chocolate.

3. COLANDER:
All fruits and vegetables (except for prewashed greens) need to be washed; keeping a colander handy makes it easy to give them a quick rinse.

4. CUTTING BOARDS (AT LEAST TWO):
Avoid damaging your countertops and cross-contaminating ingredients by always prepping produce on a cutting board. We like polypropylene plastic boards because they are sturdy, won't dull knives, and resist odors and stains. Plus, you can pop them in the dishwasher to sterilize them. Easy!

5. ICE CUBE TRAY:
Many of our recipes call for ice cubes, so make sure you always keep a full tray in the freezer.

6. JUICER:
A handheld juicer is essential for juicing fresh lemons, limes, oranges, and grapefruits. You can also use a press-style juicer or a twist-style one.

7. MEASURING CUPS AND SPOONS:
These are indispensable for measuring out the right amount of an ingredient. Winging it could result in a smoothie with too much or too little liquid.

8. SILICONE SPATULA:
It's smart to have a few different sizes of these flexible kitchen tools for scraping down the sides of your blender. Plus, a small, narrow one is ideal for getting the last bit of almond butter out of the jar.

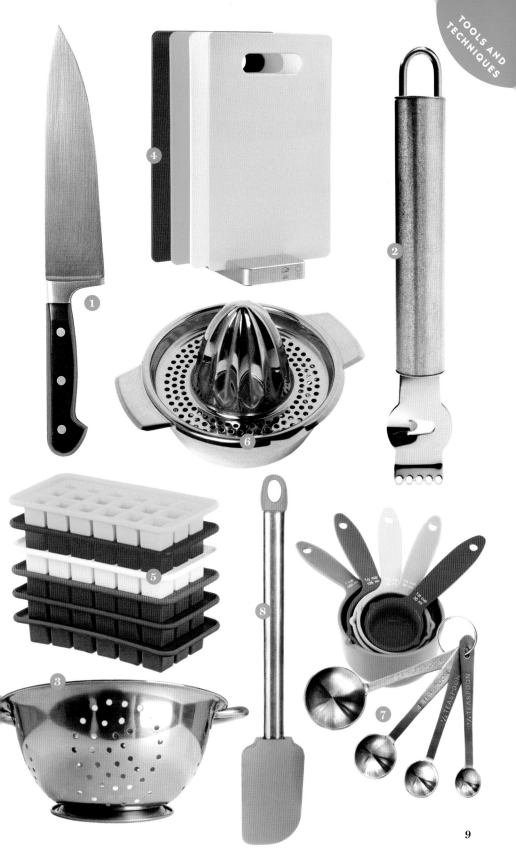

1

4

2

6

5

3

8

7

9

INGREDIENTS 101

PRODUCE

Fresh, seasonal picks are always going to be the most flavorful produce in smoothies and other recipes. If you can shop for fruits and vegetables locally, that's the best choice for the environment and your local economy. But you'll see that we also recommend using frozen fruits and vegetables in many of our recipes because the produce is picked at the peak of ripeness and flash-frozen to lock in nutrients. Plus, you can use only as much as you need and put the rest back in the freezer for your next smoothie, cutting down on waste.

ORGANIC VS. CONVENTIONAL

We definitely support organic farming, and it's great to choose organic when it fits your budget. But so many of us just aren't getting enough fruits and vegetables of any kind. In fact, a Centers for Disease Control and *Prevention* study found that just 1 in 10 Americans gets the recommended 1 ½ to 2 cups of fruit and the 2 to 3 cups of vegetables per day that are needed for long-term health. We say, just eat them—organic or conventional! And the healthy smoothies in these pages can help you reach those daily goals easily and deliciously.

WASH IT WELL

Whether the fresh produce you buy is organic and locally sourced or conventional and hauled hundreds of miles, one thing is certain—it should all be washed before eating. What's the best way? Place the produce in a colander and give it a rinse under cold running water just before using. You may want to opt for a package of triple-washed spinach or other greens for your smoothies, which don't need to be rewashed before blending—they're ready to eat.

ADD-INS

While fruits and veggies make up the majority of the ingredients in our recipes, you'll also want to keep other staples on hand.

Nut butters: almond, peanut, cashew, etc.
Milk: whole, low-fat, fat-free
Nondairy beverages: almond milk, oat milk, soy milk, etc.
Ground spices: cinnamon, ginger, nutmeg, turmeric, etc.
Orange juice
Yogurt: Greek and low-fat vanilla-flavored
Protein powder: turn to page 13 for a guide to choosing one that's right for you
Seeds: chia, hemp, and flax
Other: vanilla extract, cocoa powder
Toppings: cacao nibs, shredded coconut, granola
Sweeteners: honey, agave nectar, maple syrup, dates

NATURAL SWEETNESS

We've tried to limit the amount of added sugar we've included in each recipe. If the ingredients had enough natural sweetness from fruit, we didn't add anything else. Veggie-based smoothies sometimes need a touch of honey or a few dates to create a sippable, craveable balance. If you'd like to adjust the recipes to make the smoothies sweeter or less sweet, go for it!

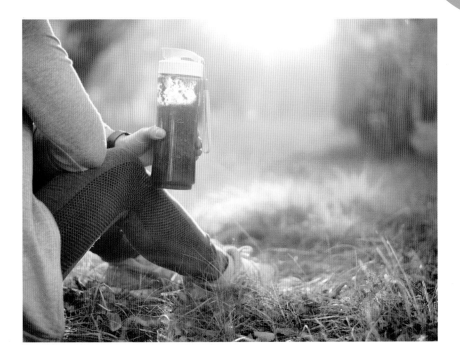

IS A SMOOTHIE A MEAL?

Americans these days are snacking as if it's their job. In the car, at the office, on the way to and from places, we're on the go and getting nutrients while we're moving. Sometimes we make up for a skipped breakfast with a couple of mid-morning snacks, or we snack through lunch because we're trying to meet a deadline. But just what makes something a snack or a meal?

Most nutritionists would define a snack as no more than 200 to 250 calories, while a meal is more in the 350- to 600-calorie range. Ideally, a snack is meant to fuel you between meals and should be just as nutrient-rich and balanced as a meal.

You'll see we've designated some of our smoothies as Breakfast (or Lunch) to Go even though they may have only about 250 calories. That's because they contain ingredients that are perfect for getting you energized and out the door. Still, they don't contain enough calories for a complete meal, so we suggest pairing them with a piece of almond butter toast, a hard-boiled egg, or a yogurt.

Some of our recipes are designed to be a snack or a drink that would accompany another meal, while others are filling enough to be a meal. If you're looking for a smoothie that offers a healthy mix of protein, fat, carbs, and fiber and is filling enough to be a meal, go for these options:

- **Gut-Health Smoothie** (page 20)

- **Health Nut Smoothie** (page 99)

- **Blueberry Cobbler Smoothie Bowl** (page 112)

- **Energy Duo Smoothie Bowl** (page 114)

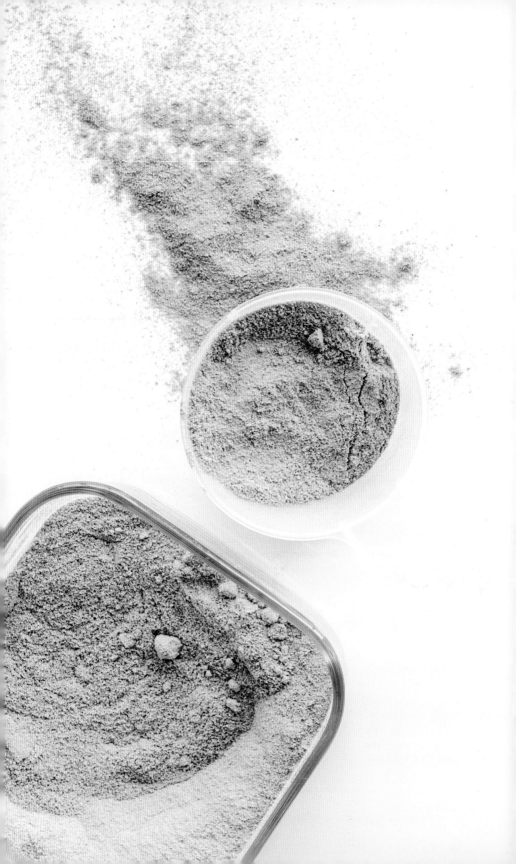

PROTEIN POWDER PICKS

You'll see protein powder used as an ingredient in many of our smoothies, but which one is the best? There are hundreds on the market, and they all sound great. The best one for you is one that meets the needs of your diet, has little or no added sugar, and tastes good. Here, we break down the most popular varieties.

WHEY PROTEIN POWDER

It's generally considered the gold standard. Whey protein is a by-product of the cheese-making process and provides substantial amounts of amino acids, the building blocks of protein. It is easy to find and blends well into smoothies, and research shows it helps build muscle when combined with strength training. It does contain lactose, so it's not appropriate for people who need to follow a dairy-free diet.

SOY PROTEIN POWDER

Soybeans contain high-quality protein and have been found to be as effective as whey protein in helping to stimulate muscle growth. In addition to being a plant-based protein, soy also contains isoflavones, which have been shown to protect against heart disease, osteoporosis, and some cancers. Isoflavones are converted by the body to phytoestrogens, which may help alleviate some symptoms of menopause, such as hot flashes. But concern over the effects of too many of these estrogen-like compounds has caused many people to avoid soy protein. If used in moderation, soy protein powder is perfectly safe, but if you already eat many other soy-based foods (milk, protein bars, etc.), you may want to opt for a different protein powder.

PEA PROTEIN POWDER

If you're avoiding both dairy and soy, plant-based pea protein may be the right fit for you. It has a pleasant, slightly grassy flavor, and most people find it easy to digest. It is deficient in the amino acid cysteine, but that doesn't mean it isn't beneficial. You'll want to vary your protein sources—a smart move anyway.

BROWN RICE PROTEIN POWDER

This powder is a plant-based, gluten-free, easily digested alternative that works well in smoothies and baked goods too. Brown rice protein is low in the amino acid lysine, so you'll want to rotate protein sources to make sure you're covering your bases.

HEMP PROTEIN POWDER

Another plant-based option, hemp may be the pick for you if you're looking to bump up the omega-3 and omega-6 fatty acids in your diet. Due to its high fat content, hemp protein powder should be stored in the refrigerator after the container is opened.

Chapter 1

Balanced Gut

We're all looking for balance in our hectic lives. It turns out that the key to that balance may lie in our gut. The term "gut" refers to our entire digestive system, and a healthy one provides our first line of immune defense. It also plays a role in staving off a number of health issues, including obesity, type 2 diabetes, heart disease, and inflammatory bowel disease. There is even a connection between our gut and our mood. For example, problems with our gastrointestinal system, such as irritable bowel syndrome (IBS), can be caused by stress. And increased anxiety can make those gut issues worse. Serotonin is the feel-good neurotransmitter, and an astounding 90 percent of serotonin receptors are found in the gut.

Unfortunately, a round of antibiotics, too much processed food, or environmental factors like a home that's too clean (really!) can throw our digestive harmony out of whack. But you can get things back on track with our gut-balancing smoothies, filled with fiber, probiotics, prebiotics (turn to page 21 for more on these), and other good-for-your-gut ingredients.

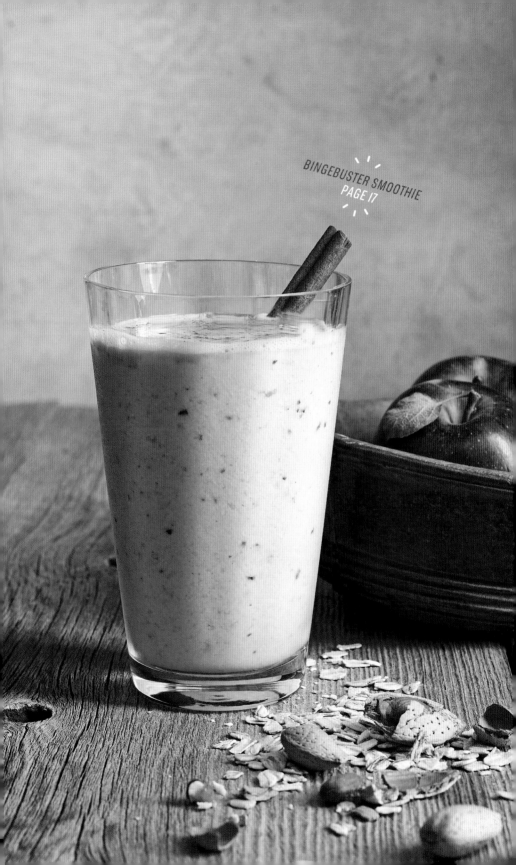

BINGEBUSTER SMOOTHIE
PAGE 17

Creamy Kale Smoothie

Total time: 5 minutes
Makes: 1 serving

→ Packed with protein and probiotics, Greek yogurt is a natural in healthy-gut smoothies. And pineapple contains bromelain, an enzyme that helps break down protein and may help reduce bloating. Together, they make this one a sweet way to be good to your gut.

INGREDIENTS

1 cup coarsely chopped kale
1½ cups frozen pineapple chunks
½ cup plain Greek yogurt
½ cup unsweetened almond milk
1 teaspoon honey

In a blender, combine kale, pineapple, yogurt, milk, and honey and blend until the mixture is smooth and frothy. Pour into 1 tall glass.

PER SERVING: 296 calories, 8.5 g fat (3 g saturated fat), 14 g protein, 143 mg sodium, 45 g carbohydrates, 36 g sugars (6 g added sugar), 5 g fiber

---

VEGAN!

Bingebuster Smoothie

Total time: 5 minutes
Makes: 1 serving

→ Stress and lack of sleep can make us want to run straight to the nearest cupcake. You can fight that urge with this fiber-packed smoothie. The apple and oats make you feel full, while the cinnamon and apple cider vinegar help stabilize blood sugar. The protein in the almond butter adds to the feeling of satiety, helping you forget all about that sugar craving (see page 19 for more on sugar).

INGREDIENTS

¾ cup unsweetened almond milk
¼ cup rolled oats
1 tablespoon almond butter
1 teaspoon apple cider vinegar
1 teaspoon ground cinnamon
1 apple, cored and chopped

In a blender, combine almond milk, oats, almond butter, apple cider vinegar, cinnamon, and apple and blend until the mixture is smooth. Pour into a tall glass.

PER SERVING: 305 calories, 13 g fat (1 g saturated fat), 7 g protein, 138 mg sodium, 45 g carbohydrates, 20 g sugars (0 g added sugar), 10 g fiber

Citrus-Pineapple Smoothie Bowl

Total time: 10 minutes
Makes: 2 servings

→ A smoothie bowl is a fun way to switch up your smoothie routine. This one features vitamin C-rich citrus fruit and heart-healthy cashews. Greek yogurt provides probiotics for a gut boost.

INGREDIENTS

FOR SMOOTHIE
½ cup fat-free Greek yogurt
½ cup frozen pineapple
   chunks
1 teaspoon vanilla extract
½ navel orange, segmented
¼ ruby red grapefruit,
   segmented

FOR TOPPING
¼ cup fat-free Greek yogurt
2 tablespoons raw cashews,
   coarsely chopped
2 tablespoons
   unsweetened shredded
   coconut
2 teaspoons chia seeds
½ navel orange, segmented
¼ ruby red grapefruit,
   segmented

1. Blend yogurt, pineapple, vanilla, orange, and grapefruit in a blender until the mixture is smooth. Divide between 2 bowls.

2. Spoon 2 tablespoons yogurt onto each smoothie bowl. Top each bowl with 1 tablespoon cashews, 1 tablespoon coconut, 1 teaspoon chia seeds, and half of the orange and grapefruit segments. Serve immediately.

PER SERVING: 240 calories, 8 g fat (4 g saturated fat), 12 g protein, 34 mg sodium, 31 g carbohydrates, 19 g sugars (0 g added sugar), 5 g fiber

 Tip Chia seeds are a nutritious addition to any smoothie, and because they expand in water, they can also help you stay hydrated throughout the day. Chia seeds are gluten-free and contain alpha-linolenic acid (ALA), which is a plant-based omega-3 fatty acid that helps fight inflammation. Store chia seeds in a sealed container in your refrigerator to keep them fresh for up to a year.

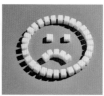

THE UGLY SIDE OF SWEETS

You're likely already trying to cut back on added sugars in your diet—not only sweeteners, but foods made with them, like desserts, drinks, cereals, crackers, and even condiments. Added sugars can contribute to weight gain and tooth decay, cause inflammation (turn to Chapter 3, page 56, for more on inflammation), and even play a role in our gut health. Consuming too much added sugar can disrupt the balance of gut microbes.

The United States Department of Agriculture's Dietary Guidelines recommend that no more than 10 percent of your total daily calories come from added sugars. For a 2,000-calorie diet, that amounts to a maximum of 200 calories, or 12 teaspoons. Currently, Americans are eating closer to 22 teaspoons of added sugar each day! It's important to note that naturally occurring sugars, like those in fruits, vegetables, and dairy products, are not considered added sugars.

Gut-Health Smoothie

Total time: 10 minutes
Makes: 1 serving

→ Maintaining a healthy gut—which is crucial for a strong immune system—requires two types of ingredients: prebiotic and probiotic (see the information at right for more gut-health basics). Prebiotic foods provide fuel for good bacteria in the gut, while probiotic foods provide the bacteria itself. This drink contains three outstanding gut-health ingredients. High in fiber, bananas and kiwifruits are prebiotic powerhouses. And kefir—similar to a liquid yogurt but with more beneficial bacteria—is a probiotic bonanza.

INGREDIENTS

1 cup chopped kale, packed
1 cup full-fat kefir
1 tablespoon creamy
   almond butter
1 frozen banana, sliced
1 kiwi, peeled

In a blender, combine kale, kefir, almond butter, banana, and kiwi and blend until the mixture is smooth. Serve in a tall glass.

PER SERVING: 436 calories, 18 g fat (6 g saturated fat), 18 g protein, 189 mg sodium, 58 g carbohydrates, 34 g sugars (0 g added sugar), 8 g fiber

GOOD GUT BUGS

Probiotics, the good bacteria that help keep our gut healthy, have gotten a ton of well-deserved attention over the past few years. They're part of our microbiome, the collection of bacteria that live both inside and outside our bodies. You can find them in fermented dairy foods, like yogurt and kefir, as well as in other fermented foods such as sauerkraut and kimchi. You can even find granola and snack bars with probiotics added to them.

Those good bacteria in our gut can be killed off when we take a round of antibiotics—and our healthy little gut tribe might not completely recover for up to a year. Other medications, like those for diabetes, blood pressure, and cancer, may also affect our microbiome.

Since a robust gut environment is vital to many aspects of our overall health, it's smart to pay attention to it and help it each day with the foods we eat. Lucky for us, smoothies are an easy way to do that!

GOOD BELLY FUEL

Prebiotics are the fuel that probiotics need in order to flourish. Prebiotics are the undigestible fiber in foods like Jerusalem artichokes, bananas, oats, asparagus, onions, leeks, apples, kiwi, soybeans, chia seeds, flaxseeds, and whole-wheat foods. Honey, maple syrup, and kombucha are also rich in prebiotics. Inulin is a naturally occurring prebiotic fiber that is also used as an added fiber in processed foods. Some people, especially those with IBS, are sensitive to inulin and other prebiotics.

If you're looking to improve your overall gut health it makes sense to focus on foods with both prebiotic and probiotic benefits. The Gut-Health Smoothie (at left) is perfect for getting everything you need in one delicious glass.

HOW TO FREEZE BANANAS:

1. Peel several ripe bananas (ripe ones are sweeter).

2. Slice into 1-inch rounds. Place banana rounds in a single layer on a parchment-lined baking sheet.

3. Freeze for two hours, until solid.

4. Transfer bananas to a zip-top freezer bag and keep in the freezer for up to six months.

RIPENING TIPS

Your bunch of bananas is looking far more green than yellow, but you'd like to use them soon. You can speed up the ripening process by doing the following:

- Place the bananas in a brown paper bag. This helps trap the ethylene gas the bananas emit. Ethylene helps the bananas convert their starch to sugars and allows the fruit to soften and change color. Adding another fruit that also releases ethylene, such as a tomato or apple, will further speed the ripening.

- Move your bananas to a warm location, such as on top of the refrigerator, on top of a warm oven, or near a radiator.

- If you're simply out of time and need to speed-ripen them, try this: Arrange the unpeeled bananas on a baking sheet and place in a 300°F oven for five to seven minutes. The bananas are ready to eat or use when the skins have turned black.

Banana-Berry Smoothie Bowl

Total time: 10 minutes
Makes: 2 servings

→ Sweet strawberries add a pink hue to this smoothie bowl, but it's not just a pretty dish. The flaxseeds add ALA, which provides antioxidants and helps block the growth of certain cancers. Plus, flaxseeds help lower cholesterol levels and relieve constipation.

PROTEIN-PACKED!

INGREDIENTS

FOR SMOOTHIE
1 cup frozen strawberries
½ cup fat-free Greek yogurt
¼ cup rolled oats
2 tablespoons water
1 tablespoon flaxseed
½ banana

FOR TOPPING
¼ cup fresh strawberries, sliced
2 tablespoons pistachios, roughly chopped
2 tablespoons unsweetened coconut
1 teaspoon chia seeds
1 teaspoon flaxseed
½ banana, sliced

1. Blend frozen strawberries, yogurt, oats, water, flaxseeds, and banana in a blender until the mixture is smooth. Divide between two bowls.

2. Top each bowl with 2 tablespoons sliced strawberries, 1 tablespoon chopped pistachios, 1 tablespoon coconut, ½ teaspoon chia seeds, ½ teaspoon flaxseeds, and half of the banana slices. Serve immediately.

PER SERVING:
278 calories, 11 g fat (4 g saturated fat), 12 g protein, 27 mg sodium, 36 g carbohydrates, 15 g sugars (0 g added sugar), 8 g fiber

Tip You can use either whole flaxseed or ground flaxseed in this recipe. Either way, store it in the refrigerator to keep it fresh longer; ground flaxseed will last for six months and whole seeds will last for a year. It makes a healthy addition to baked goods too.

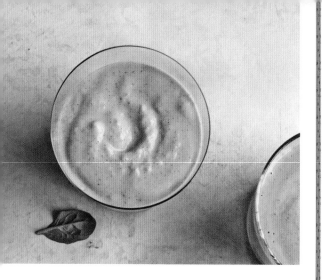

Pear-Spinach Smoothie

Total time: 10 minutes
Makes: 1 serving

→ Need to get things moving? Probiotic-rich yogurt can help keep you regular. And one medium pear boasts nearly 6 grams of fiber, making it a go-to ingredient when you need to go.

INGREDIENTS
1 cup spinach
¾ cup Greek yogurt
1 Bartlett pear, quartered
½-inch piece fresh ginger, peeled and grated
Handful of ice

Add spinach, yogurt, pear, ginger, and ice to a blender and blend until the mixture is smooth. Serve in a tall glass.

PER SERVING: 306 calories, 10 g fat (4.5 g saturated fat), 19 g protein, 91 mg sodium, 36 g carbohydrates, 25 g sugars (0 g added sugar), 6 g fiber

> *Tip* **Not sure how to pick a ripe pear? Apply gentle pressure to the neck (the top area by the stem) with your thumb. If it yields slightly to pressure, it's ripe and ready to eat. Not soft enough? Give it another day or so at room temperature. Placing it in a brown paper bag helps speed ripening.**

VEGAN & FIBER-PACKED!

Fruity Green Smoothie

Total time: 10 minutes
Makes: 2 servings

→ Talk about fully loaded with goodness! Five varieties of fruit plus spinach, celery, and cucumber add up to a smoothie that delivers more than a third of your daily fiber requirement. And pectin, the soluble prebiotic fiber in apples, has been found to increase butyrate, a fatty acid that feeds good gut bacteria.

INGREDIENTS
2 cups water
½ cup baby spinach
2 stalks celery, chopped
1 Bartlett pear, chopped
1 green apple, chopped
1 ripe banana (preferably frozen), sliced
2 slices ripe mango
¼ cup diced pineapple
¼ English (seedless) cucumber, sliced
1 teaspoon honey

In a blender, combine water, spinach, celery, pear, apple, banana, mango, pineapple, cucumber, and honey and blend until the mixture is smooth. Serve in 2 tall glasses.

PER SERVING: 217 calories, 1 g fat (0 g saturated fat), 3 g protein, 46 mg sodium, 53 g carbohydrates, 35 g sugars (3 g added sugar), 9 g fiber

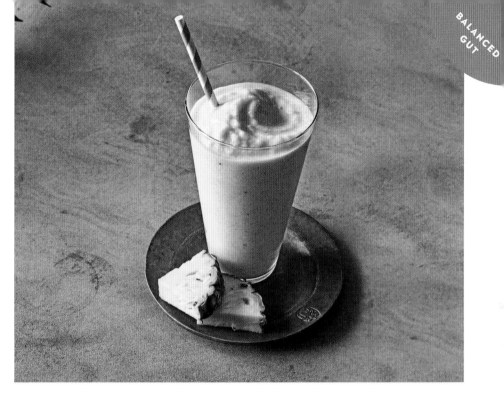

Caribbean Dream Smoothie

Total time: 5 minutes
Makes: 1 serving

→ If you're plagued by a nervous stomach before big events, try sipping this smoothie beforehand. It includes banana, which contains the relaxing mineral magnesium. Yogurt boasts probiotics that may ease anxiety. Plus, the bromelain in pineapple facilitates digestion.

INGREDIENTS

½ cup pineapple chunks
¼ cup 2 percent Greek yogurt
¼ cup refrigerated unsweetened coconut milk
¼ cup orange juice
¼ large banana
Handful of ice

1. Blend pineapple, yogurt, coconut milk, orange juice, banana, and ice until smooth.

2. Serve in a tall glass. For best results, sip 2 hours before you need to calm your nerves.

PER SERVING: 156 calories, 3 g fat (2 g saturated fat), 6 g protein, 32 mg sodium, 29 g carbohydrate, 21 g sugars (1.5 g added sugar), 2 g fiber

Tip Prep the ingredients the night before so you can jump out of bed and blend. If you have a personal blender, you can store the ingredients in the to-go blending cup. If you have a traditional blender, simply add all the ingredients (except ice) to an airtight plastic container and store it in the fridge overnight.

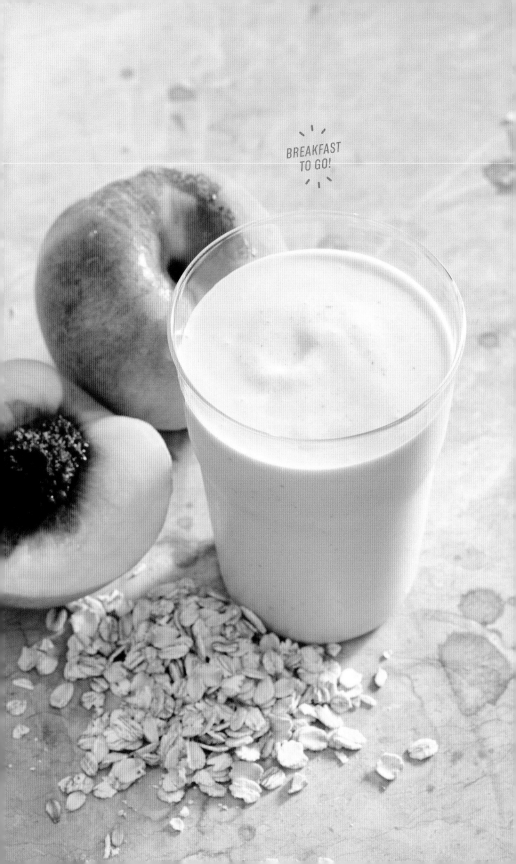

Peaches & Cream Oatmeal Smoothie

Total time: 5 minutes
Makes: 2 servings

➜ No time for a leisurely meal? Grab this probiotic-rich take on morning oatmeal and go. Whole-grain oats contain prebiotic fiber that promotes gut health (see photo at left).

INGREDIENTS
½ cup whole milk
½ cup plain whole-milk
  Greek yogurt
½ cup rolled oats
1 cup frozen peaches
½ frozen banana
½ cup ice

Blend milk, yogurt, oats, peaches, banana, and ice until smooth. Serve in 2 tall glasses.

PER SERVING: 217 calories,
 5.5 g fat (2.5 g saturated fat),
11 g protein, 47 mg sodium,
33 g carbohydrates, 15 g sugars
(0 g added sugar), 4 g fiber

Tip Oats not only add a boost for your digestion, but they also help you feel more full thanks to the fiber and resistant starch they contain.

Tropical Mango Smoothie

Total time: 10 minutes
Makes: 1 serving

➜ Ginger has long been used in traditional medicine to help alleviate upset stomach and nausea, and there's scientific evidence to back that up. Blend this tropical treat when your belly isn't quite right and you'll be feeling like yourself in no time.

INGREDIENTS
½ cup unsweetened
  pineapple juice, chilled
1 cup diced fresh mango
1 banana, sliced
2 teaspoons fresh lime juice
½ teaspoon grated, peeled
  fresh ginger
3 ice cubes

In a blender, combine pineapple juice, mango, banana, lime juice, ginger, and ice and blend until the mixture is smooth. Serve in a tall glass.

PER SERVING: 274 calories,
1 g fat (0.5 g saturated fat),
3 g protein, 6 mg sodium,
69 g carbohydrates, 46 g sugars
(0 g added sugar), 6 g fiber

Tip The color of a mango doesn't indicate ripeness. Go by the feel instead. A ripe mango will yield slightly to gentle pressure, and the stem end should have a fruity aroma.

Carrot-Coconut Smoothie

VEGAN!

Total time: 5 minutes
Makes: 1 serving

➜ The flavors in this energizing smoothie will remind you of carrot cake—but without all the added sugar! With 30 percent of the fiber you need for the day, your gut will be as pleased as your taste buds.

INGREDIENTS
1 cup freshly grated peeled carrots
1 cup frozen pineapple chunks
1 small apple, preferably McIntosh or Gala, peeled and diced
¼ cup refrigerated unsweetened coconut milk
Pinch of ground cinnamon

In a blender, combine carrots, pineapple, apple, coconut milk, and cinnamon and blend until the mixture is smooth. Serve in a tall glass.

PER SERVING: 210 calories, 2 g fat (1 g saturated fat), 2 g protein, 89 mg sodium, 51 g carbohydrates, 36 g sugars (1.5 g added sugar), 7 g fiber

Tip Not enough time to grate carrots? You can find pre-grated carrots in the refrigerated section of the produce aisle.

Avocado & Kiwi Smoothie

Total time: 10 minutes
Makes: 2 servings

➜ Though it's known for its creamy texture, an avocado is actually a great source of fiber. One fruit contains 9 grams! Pair that with fiber-rich kiwi and pineapple and you've got a recipe for a super-filling, gut-friendly breakfast or snack.

INGREDIENTS
1 avocado
2 kiwifruits, peeled and quartered
1 cup plain fat-free yogurt
1 ½ cups frozen pineapple chunks

In a blender, combine avocado, kiwifruit, yogurt, and pineapple and blend until the mixture is smooth. Serve in 2 tall glasses.

PER SERVING: 341 calories, 15 g fat (2 g saturated fat), 11 g protein, 103 mg sodium, 14 g carbohydrates, 28 g sugars (0 g added sugar), 11 g fiber

Tip Benefit from an added dose of fiber by leaving the kiwi's furry skin on. Simply rinse it well and throw the entire fruit into the blender! Eating the skin will up the fiber content in this smoothie by more than 30 percent.

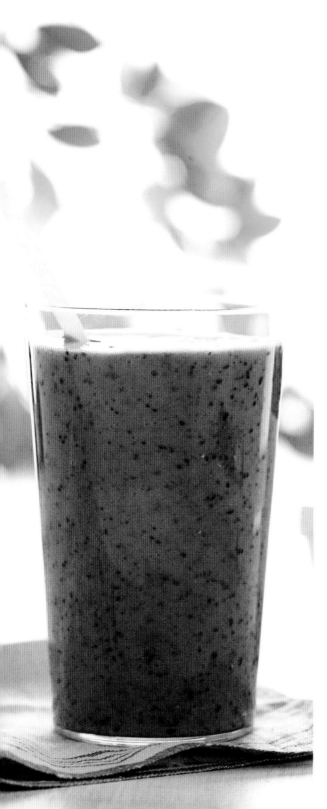

BRUNCH PICK!

Berry-Banana Smoothie

Total time: 10 minutes
Makes: 4 servings

→ Oats add body to your smoothies, and the resistant starch this whole grain contains helps you feel fuller longer. Another bonus of resistant starch? It causes less gas than other fibers.

INGREDIENTS

2 cups frozen strawberries
1 cup vanilla low-fat yogurt
1 banana, sliced
½ cup rolled oats
½ cup orange juice
1 tablespoon honey

In a blender, combine strawberries, yogurt, banana, oats, orange juice, and honey. Blend until the mixture is smooth. Serve in 4 glasses.

PER SERVING: 171 calories, 2 g fat (1 g saturated fat), 5 g protein, 43 mg sodium, 36 g carbohydrates, 23 g sugars (4.5 g added sugar), 3.5 g fiber

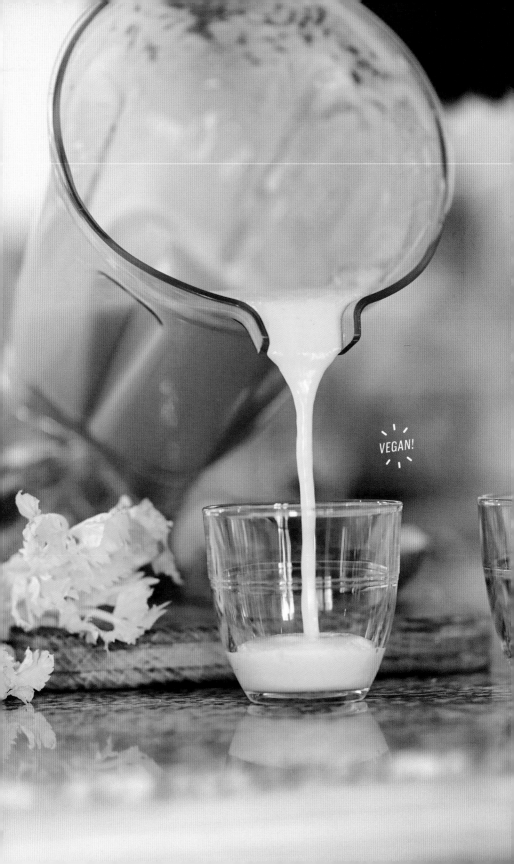

VEGAN!

"Milk" & Honey Smoothie

Total time: 5 minutes
Makes: 2 servings

→ Make use of the celery lingering in your produce drawer with this blender juice that combines it with almond milk, cucumber, and grapes for a sip-worthy snack. Celery has anti-inflammatory benefits and helps digestion with both its high water content and its fiber. Celery (including the stalk, leaves, and seeds) has been used in traditional medicine for centuries to treat stomach problems and joint issues and has even been used as a libido stimulant.

INGREDIENTS
1 ½ cups unsweetened
   almond milk
1 medium Kirby cucumber,
   peeled and sliced
1 cup seedless green
   grapes
2 medium stalks celery,
   peeled and sliced
1 tablespoon honey

In a blender, combine almond milk, cucumber, grapes, celery, and honey. Blend until the mixture is smooth. Serve in 2 tall glasses.

PER SERVING: 124 calories, 2 g fat (0 g saturated fat), 2 g protein, 170 mg sodium, 26 g carbohydrates, 21 g sugars (9 g added sugar), 2 g fiber

 You can swap out the almond milk for other options like regular milk, soy milk, oat milk, or coconut milk.

FIBER-PACKED!

Blueberry-Orange Jump-Start Smoothie

Total time: 5 minutes
Makes: 2 servings

→ Lost your mojo? The zingy flavor of ginger gives you the kick you need to get your day started. And the berries provide a healthy hit of fiber, so you'll feel full until lunch.

INGREDIENTS
1 cup frozen strawberries
½ cup fresh blueberries
½ cup fresh orange juice
2 teaspoons grated, peeled
   fresh ginger
¼ cup plain low-fat yogurt
2 ice cubes

In a blender, combine strawberries, blueberries, orange juice, ginger, yogurt, and ice cubes and blend until the mixture is smooth. Serve in 2 tall glasses.

PER SERVING: 96 calories, 1 g fat (0.5 g saturated fat), 3 g protein, 24 mg sodium, 21 g carbohydrates, 14 g sugars (0 g added sugar), 3 g fiber

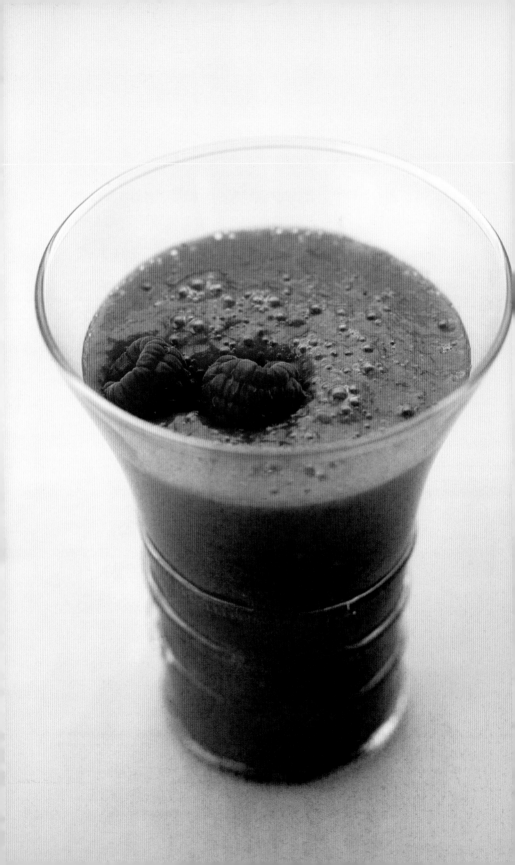

Spring in a Glass VEGAN!

Total time: 10 minutes
Makes: 2 servings

→ Rhubarb is a spring ingredient that pairs perfectly with sweet raspberries. It offers fiber and supplies as much potassium as a cup of milk, while raspberries ramp up the gut-health factor in this pretty blush drink. One cup of the berries has an impressive 8 grams of fiber, which acts as a prebiotic (see page 21), helping your belly's good bacteria thrive.

INGREDIENTS

2 medium stalks rhubarb, sliced; or 1 ½ cups frozen chopped rhubarb
1 tablespoon honey
1 (6 ounce) container fresh raspberries
1 cup cold water
1 cup ice cubes
1 small (½ inch) piece fresh peeled ginger, sliced (see ginger storage tip, below)

1. In a blender, combine rhubarb, honey, raspberries, water, ice, and ginger. Blend until the mixture is smooth.

2. Strain and pour into 2 tall glasses.

PER SERVING: 148 calories, 1 g fat (0 g saturated fat), 2 g protein, 4 mg sodium, 21 g carbohydrates, 13 g sugars (9 g added sugar), 6.5 g fiber

Tip To store fresh ginger in the refrigerator, wrap it in a paper towel, then tightly in plastic wrap. It will stay fresh for up to two weeks.

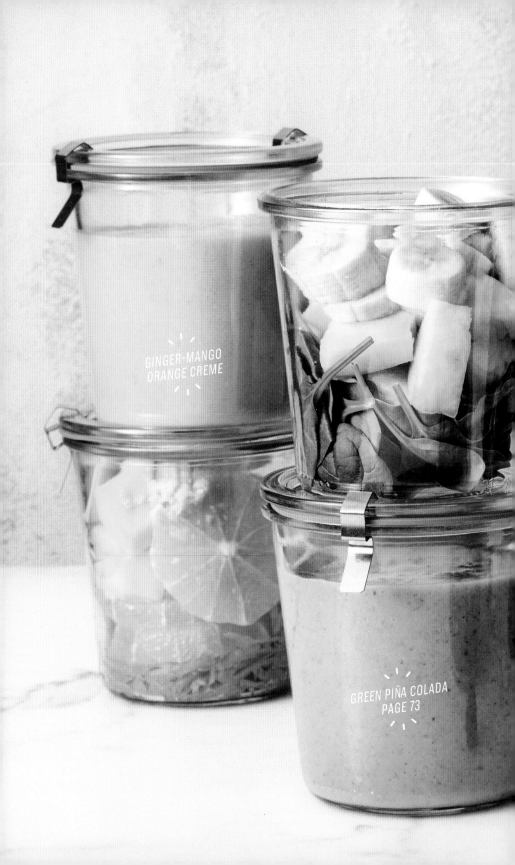

GINGER-MANGO
ORANGE CREME

GREEN PIÑA COLADA
PAGE 73

Ginger-Mango Orange Creme

Total time: 5 minutes, plus freezing time
Makes: 2 servings

→ The soothing benefits of ginger combine with probiotic-packed yogurt for a gut-healthy shake. Freeze the fruits and veggies overnight in a freezer-safe bag. They'll be ready to blend up with the juice and yogurt whenever you need them.

MEAL-PREP IDEA!

INGREDIENTS

FREEZE

1 cup mango chunks
1 small orange, peeled and seeded
1 medium carrot, grated (about ½ cup)
1 teaspoon grated fresh ginger

ADD

1 cup orange-carrot juice
½ cup vanilla yogurt

1. Place mango, orange, carrot, and ginger in a zip-top plastic bag or freezer-safe jar. Freeze overnight or longer.

2. When ready to prepare, add juice and yogurt to a blender, then add frozen ingredients. Blend until smooth. Serve in 2 tall glasses.

PER SERVING: 195 calories, 1 g fat (0.5 g saturated fat), 5 g protein, 110 mg sodium, 43 g carbohydrates, 37 g sugars (5 g added sugar), 4 g fiber

BERRY, CHIA & MINT SMOOTHIE
PAGE 44

Chapter 2

Glowing Skin

S kin. It's one of the first things people notice when they meet you. It's also the largest organ in our bodies, which means it deserves some serious attention. And while what we put on our skin certainly matters, what we put inside our bodies counts just as much when it comes to our skin's appearance.

Luckily, ingredients that can make your smoothie taste delicious, like mangoes, carrots, peaches, and berries, can also give your skin an inner glow. Nutrients like beta-carotene, vitamins C and E, and ingredients such as collagen have been shown to help fight the effects of aging on our skin and can even help protect it from the sun's harmful rays. Glow getters, it's time to schedule an appointment with your blender ASAP!

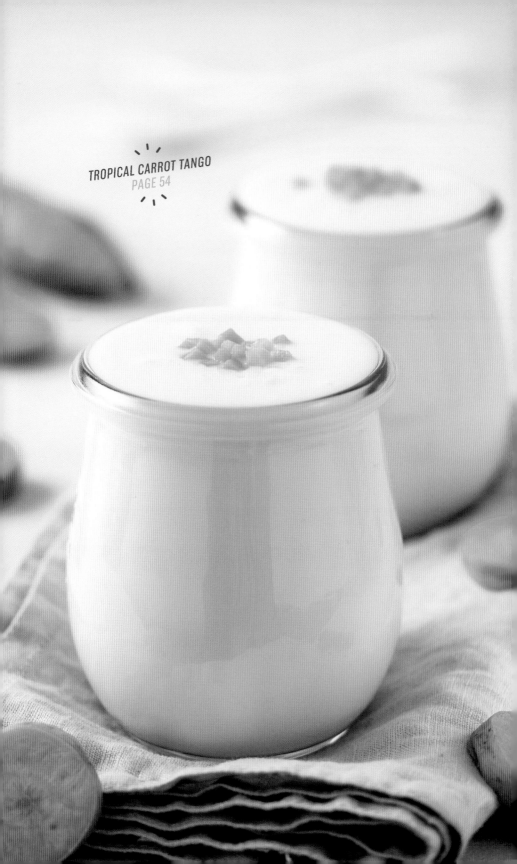

TROPICAL CARROT TANGO
PAGE 54

Papaya Punch

VEGAN!

Total time: 10 minutes
Makes: 1 serving

→ Papayas are loaded with the carotenoids beta-carotene and lycopene. Beta-carotene is a precursor to vitamin A, which is needed for skin and eye cell growth, as well as a healthy immune and reproductive system. A study in PLOS ONE found that just three more servings a day can measurably improve your skin's appearance, reducing redness and imparting a healthy glow. All the more reason to blend up this beauty!

INGREDIENTS

1 cup papaya nectar or orange juice, chilled
1 cup diced fresh papaya
1 tablespoon fresh lime juice
1 drop coconut extract (optional)
3 ice cubes

In a blender, combine papaya nectar or orange juice, papaya, lime juice, coconut extract (if using), and ice cubes and blend until the mixture is smooth. Serve in a tall glass.

PER SERVING: 209 calories, 1 g fat (0 g saturated fat), 1 g protein, 24 mg sodium, 53 g carbohydrates, 46 g sugars (15 g added sugar), 4 g fiber

Tip If you've never prepared papaya before, this tropical fruit can be a little intimidating. Choose a papaya that is soft to the touch (but not mushy). The outside color can vary from yellow to green, depending on the variety. If you have to buy an unripe papaya, you can ripen it on the counter for a few days. When it's ripe, slice the fruit in half lengthwise and remove and discard the black seeds. You can then scoop out the melon-colored flesh with a large spoon or cut it into slices with a knife.

Green Thumb Smoothie

VEGAN!

Total time: 10 minutes
Makes: 1 serving

→ This hydrating sparkler tastes as if it came straight from the garden. And studies on mice show that grapes may protect skin from cancer caused by UVB light from the sun. (Human studies are in the works.)

INGREDIENTS

½ cup sparkling water, chilled
1 cup frozen seedless green grapes
1 cup seeded, diced cucumber

In a blender, combine sparkling water, grapes, and cucumber and blend until the mixture is smooth. Serve in a tall glass.

PER SERVING: 120 calories, 0.5 g fat (0 g saturated fat), 2 g protein, 21 mg sodium, 30 g carbohydrate, 25 g sugars (0 g added sugar), 2 g fiber

Green Goddess Smoothie

Total time: 10 minutes
Makes: 2 servings

→ Hydration—check. Nearly 100 percent of your vitamin C needs for the day—check. Healthy, skin-plumping fats—check. This gorgeous green drink blends naturally sweet fruits and vitamin-rich veggies for a great-tasting, skin-perfecting refresher.

INGREDIENTS

1 cup baby spinach
1 cup cucumber chunks
½ avocado, pitted and peeled
1 large kiwifruit, peeled and chopped
½ cup plain kefir, chilled
½ cup fresh orange juice
¼ cup fresh mint leaves

In a blender, combine spinach, cucumber, avocado, kiwifruit, kefir, orange juice, and mint leaves and blend until the mixture is smooth. Serve in 2 tall glasses.

PER SERVING: 186 calories, 8.5 g fat (1.5 g saturated fat), 6 g protein, 55 mg sodium, 25 g carbohydrates, 15 g sugars (0 g added sugar), 7 g fiber

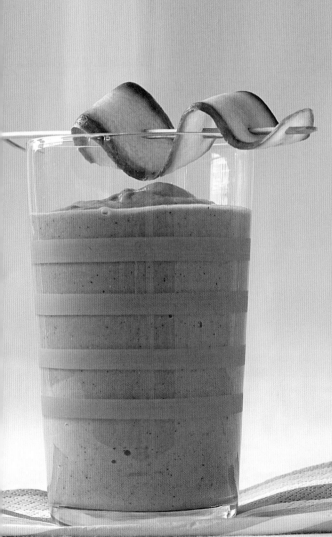

Tip **Make fresh herbs last longer** by storing them properly. Trim the stems, then place in a water-filled jar. Cover the leafy portion of the herbs with a small plastic bag and store the jar in the fridge. Change the water daily.

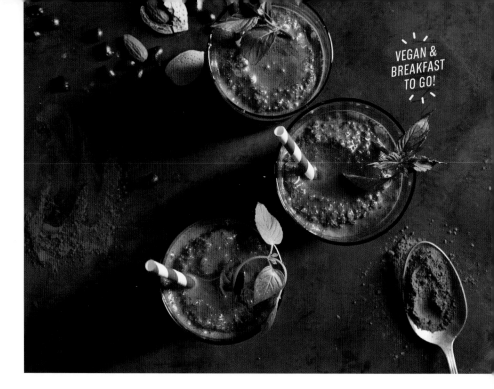

VEGAN & BREAKFAST TO GO!

Magic De-Puffer Smoothie

Total time: 5 minutes
Makes: 2 servings

→ A vacation or work travel can result in eating saltier food than usual or drinking more booze than you normally do. This can leave you with puffy eyes and a general feeling of being bloated. You can look and feel better quickly with this Magic De-Puffer Smoothie. Potassium-rich bananas counteract the puffing effects of excess sodium, while coffee, a natural diuretic, helps flush fluid. Almond butter adds a dose of satiating fiber and protein to help you get back in balance.

INGREDIENTS
½ cup refrigerated unsweetened almond milk
½ cup coffee, chilled
2 tablespoons almond butter
2 tablespoons unsweetened cocoa powder
¼–½ teaspoon peppermint extract
1 frozen banana

In a blender, combine almond milk, coffee, almond butter, cocoa powder, peppermint extract, and banana until the mixture is smooth and frothy. Serve in 2 glasses.

PER SERVING:
77 calories, 11 g fat (1 g saturated fat), 5 g protein, 49 mg sodium, 20 g carbohydrates, 8 g sugars (0 g added sugar), 5 g fiber

Tip **Keep your cocoa powder fresh by storing it in an airtight container in a cool, dark place. Do not store cocoa powder in the fridge, as the humidity may cause it to spoil.**

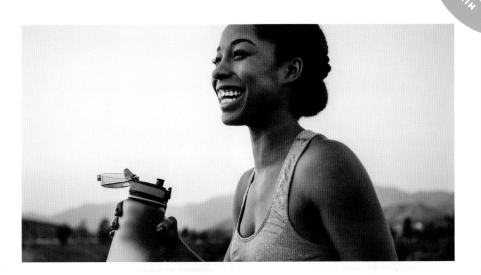

YOUR SKIN DE-PUFFING CHECKLIST

Maybe you had a few too many margaritas along with your Mexican food, or you stayed up late with girlfriends watching rom-coms and eating salty popcorn. Or perhaps you're dealing with monthly period-related water retention. Whatever the reason, you woke up looking and feeling bloated, and you need to fix things stat! Check out our de-puffing checklist and start feeling like yourself soon.

DOS

☑ **Water.** Drink at least eight 8-ounce glasses each day, plus more if you're active. It might sound counterintuitive to drink water when you're feeling puffy, but it will help transport that extra sodium out of your body.

☑ **Caffeine.** It's a diuretic, so it can help reduce minor swelling.

☑ **Potassium.** If you're bloated due to too much sodium, this electrolyte will help rebalance your sodium levels. Sodium holds on to water in the skin, making you appear bloated.

☑ **Go low-sodium.** You'll want to avoid super-salty foods for the next few days. Skip the chips, soups, packaged and processed foods, and restaurant food.

☑ **Natural diuretics.** Cucumber contains caffeic acid, which fights swelling. Celery helps balance your electrolytes. These vegetables, along with watercress, artichoke, and asparagus, are all-natural diuretics.

☑ **Sweat it out.** Even a short burst of cardio will help you get rid of excess sodium and feel better faster.

DON'TS

☒ **Alcohol.** Avoid it for a few days or you'll be right back in Puffytown.

☒ **Salty and processed food.** Stick to fruits, veggies, and other whole foods to look and feel your best.

Pumpkin Detox Smoothie

Total time: 5 minutes
Makes: 1 serving

➜ We think of pumpkin as a flavorful fall ingredient, but it has skin-saving benefits we can use all year long. Just like the other orange-fleshed ingredients in this chapter (papaya, carrots, apricots, etc.), pumpkin is rich in beta-carotene, along with lutein and zeaxanthin, which help protect our eyes and skin from the sun.

INGREDIENTS
½ cup canned pumpkin puree
½ cup milk of your choice
¼ cup plain whole-milk Greek yogurt
1 medium orange, peeled
¼ teaspoon pumpkin pie spice
Handful of ice

In a blender, combine pumpkin, milk, yogurt, orange, pumpkin pie spice, and ice until the mixture is smooth. Serve in a glass.

PER SERVING (using whole milk): 249 calories, 8 g fat (4 g saturated fat), 12 g protein, 80 mg sodium, 34 g carbohydrates, 26 g sugars (0 g added sugar), 6 g fiber

Tip Since you'll be using only ½ cup of pumpkin puree in this recipe, save the rest of the can to make moist muffins and banana bread. Pumpkin puree will keep in the refrigerator in an airtight container for up to three days.

BREAKFAST TO GO!

Silky Skin Smoothie

Total time: 5 minutes
Makes: 1 serving

→ Apricots and carrots are rich in the antioxidant beta-carotene, which the body converts into vitamin A. The vitamin can potentially offset skin aging, as well as damage from environmental factors like UV rays and pollution. This smoothie also contains cinnamon, which can improve circulation, helping skin repair itself.

INGREDIENTS
½ cup ice cubes
⅓ cup whole-milk Greek yogurt
¼ cup grated carrot
1 teaspoon honey
½ teaspoon ground cinnamon
2 dried apricot halves, chopped
1 fresh apricot, pitted and coarsely chopped

In a blender, combine ice, yogurt, carrot, honey, cinnamon, dried apricots, and fresh apricot and blend until the mixture is smooth. Serve in a glass.

PER SERVING: 130 calories, 3.5 g fat (2 g saturated fat), 8 g protein, 49 mg sodium, 21 g carbohydrates, 17 g sugars (6 g added sugar), 3 g fiber

Berry, Chia & Mint Smoothie

Total time: 10 minutes
Makes: 2 servings

→ One cup of strawberries contains more than 100 percent of your daily vitamin C needs. Vitamin C aids in collagen production, which helps your skin retain its youthful glow. And this smoothie can also fight food waste. When your berries look as if they're on their way out, throw them in a freezer bag with the other ingredients, where they'll be waiting until you're ready to blend them up.

INGREDIENTS

FREEZE

1 cup sliced strawberries
½ cup raspberries
½ cup grated beet
(from 1 medium beet)
⅓ cup mint leaves
1 tablespoon chia seeds

ADD
1 cup unsweetened
almond milk

1. Place berries, beet, mint, and chia seeds in a zip-top plastic bag or freezer-safe jar. Freeze overnight or longer.

2. When ready to prepare, add almond milk to a blender, then add frozen ingredients. Blend until smooth. Serve in 2 tall glasses.

PER SERVING: 105 calories, 3.5 g fat (0.5 g saturated fat), 3 g protein, 115 mg sodium, 17 g carbohydrates, 7 g sugars (0 g added sugar), 8 g fiber

Stress-Less Smoothie

Total time: 5 minutes
Makes: 1 serving

→ The stress hormone cortisol can trigger a breakout, cause redness, or even delay a wound's healing. This calming drink is made with kefir, an ingredient packed with probiotics (see page 21) that may help ease anxiety and trigger the release of serotonin. Berries and peaches provide vitamin C, a potential cortisol cutter, while hemp seeds deliver magnesium, which can help relax the mind and muscles.

INGREDIENTS
½ cup plain full-fat kefir, chilled
½ cup raspberries
1 tablespoon hemp seeds
1 peach, pitted and sliced
Handful of ice

In a blender, combine kefir, raspberries, hemp seeds, peach, and ice. Blend until the mixture is smooth. Serve in a glass.

PER SERVING: 221 calories, 9 g fat (3 g saturated fat), 9 g protein, 54 mg sodium, 29 g carbohydrates, 21 g sugars (0 g added sugar), 6 g fiber

Tip If you don't have hemp seeds on hand, add a tablespoon of almond butter instead for a comparable magnesium boost.

CALCIUM BOOST!

Sun Shake

Total time: 5 minutes
Makes: 1 serving

→ Certain foods act like SPF in different ways: Green tea contains catechin antioxidants, which have been shown to enhance DNA repair and reduce skin cancer risk, while carrots and mangoes pack beta-carotene and vitamin C, which may prevent UV-induced damage. Chia seeds have omega-3s that help keep skin moisturized, preventing dryness that comes with sun exposure. This shake combines all these ingredients in one delicious pre-beach treat. Sip before heading out into the sun, but you'll still want to slather on the SPF and wear a wide-brimmed hat.

VEGAN!

INGREDIENTS

1 cup frozen mango cubes
½ cup refrigerated unsweetened coconut milk
½ cup green tea, chilled
1 tablespoon protein powder (see page 13 for a guide to picking protein powder)
1 tablespoon chia seeds
1 tablespoon ground ginger
2 carrots, peeled and chopped
Handful of ice

In a blender, combine mango, coconut milk, green tea, protein powder, chia seeds, ginger, carrots, and ice until the mixture is smooth. Serve in a glass.

PER SERVING: 308 calories, 7 g fat (3 g saturated fat), 11 g protein, 194 mg sodium, 56 g carbohydrates, 37 g sugars (3 g added sugar), 12 g fiber

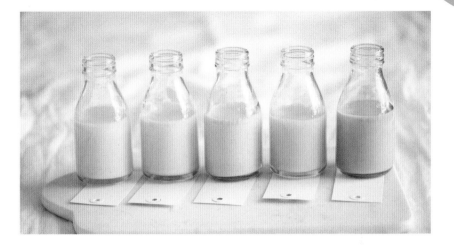

NO-MOO MILK OPTIONS

There are so many alternative nondairy milks (or mylks) these days, it can make your head spin. We've broken down the differences here. Regular cow's milk is great too (and is the best source of calcium), but if you're looking for one that's nondairy, this handy guide will help you choose. One thing to note: The "original" flavor of most alternative milk is sweetened, so be sure to look for the unsweetened varieties.

	Other nutrients	Calories	Fat	Protein	Carbs	Fiber	Calcium
Soy milk	Potassium, B vitamins	80	4 g	7 g	3 g	2 g	300 mg
Rice milk	Vitamins D, B12	120	2.5 g	1 g	23 g	0 g	300 mg
Pea milk	Vitamin D, iron	70	4.5 g	8 g	0 g	0 g	450 mg
Oat milk	Potassium, B vitamins	120	5 g	3 g	16 g	1 g	350 mg
Almond milk	Potassium	30	2.5 g	1 g	1 g	1 g	450 mg
Cashew milk	Potassium	50	4 g	1 g	2 g	0 g	47 mg
Coconut milk	Vitamins E and A	40	4 g	0 g	1 g	0 g	460 mg
Hemp milk	Iron, magnesium	60	4.5 g	3 g	0 g	0 g	257 mg

Per 8-ounce serving (for unsweetened, unflavored nondairy beverages; amounts can vary by brand)

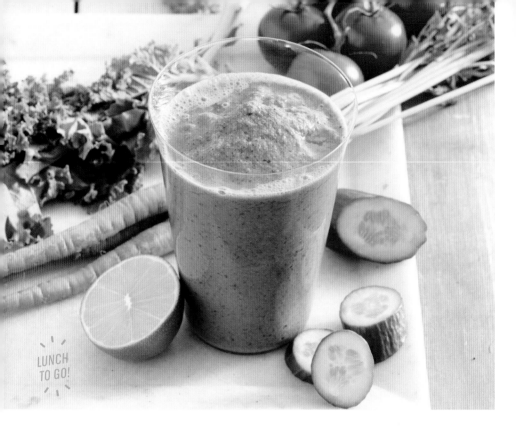

LUNCH TO GO!

Tomato-Kale Gazpacho Smoothie

Total time: 5 minutes
Makes: 2 servings

→ It's hard to believe, but just 1 in 10 of us is eating enough veggies. Lack of time and cooking knowledge can be an obstacle for lots of people. Make it easy to get the nutrients your skin needs with this veggie-packed smoothie. With five different vegetables in one glass, this can stand in for a whole salad—fast. Pair it up with lean protein for a complete meal.

INGREDIENTS

¼ cup water
2 tablespoons fresh lime juice
½ cup plain Greek yogurt
¼ teaspoon ground cumin
2 large kale leaves, stems removed
1 cup fresh or canned diced tomatoes
1 small carrot, peeled and chopped
1 small English cucumber, chopped
½ stalk celery, chopped
Hot sauce, to taste (optional)
½ cup ice

In a blender, combine water, lime juice, yogurt, cumin, kale, tomatoes, carrot, cucumber, celery, hot sauce (if using), and ice. Blend until the mixture is smooth. Serve in 2 glasses.

PER SERVING: 112 calories, 2.5 g fat (1.5 g saturated fat), 8 g protein, 379 mg sodium, 16 g carbohydrates, 8 g sugars (0 g added sugar), 3 g fiber

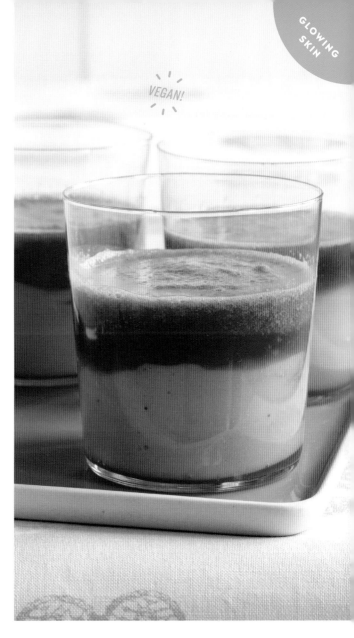

VEGAN!

Sunrise Smoothie

Total time: 5 minutes
Makes: 2 servings

➜ Don't toss out fruits when they start to get mushy—that's when antioxidant levels peak (and taste is often sweetest). And speaking of antioxidants, fresh ginger is loaded with them, which can reduce skin redness and irritation. Plus, hydrating watermelon (it's 92 percent water) helps keep skin looking its best and contains high levels of the antioxidant lycopene, which protects skin from the sun's harmful rays.

INGREDIENTS

1 cup mango chunks
½ banana, sliced
1 teaspoon fresh lime juice
¼ teaspoon grated, peeled fresh ginger
1 ice cube
1 teaspoon honey
2 cups seedless watermelon chunks

1. In a blender, combine mango, banana, lime juice, ginger, ice cube, and honey and blend until the mixture is smooth and frothy.

2. Divide evenly between 2 glasses; rinse blender.

3. Blend watermelon and pour evenly over the mango layer in each glass.

PER SERVING: 138 calories, 0 g fat (0 g saturated fat), 1.5 g protein, 5.5 mg sodium, 39 g carbohydrates, 33 g sugars (3 g added sugar), 4 g fiber

Strawberry & Apricot Smoothie

Total time: 5 minutes
Makes: 2 servings

→ This morning blend is already packed with collagen-boosting vitamin C from the strawberries, but if you're looking for a protein-rich beauty aid, add a handful of almonds. Almonds contain the antioxidant vitamin E, which helps protect the skin from the damaging effects of environmental free radicals produced by exposure to the sun, air pollution, and cigarette smoke. Almonds are also the richest source of vitamin E of all nuts.

Tip **Love strawberries? Save money** and buy a large bag of frozen ones to keep on hand for this recipe and other morning smoothies. Use what you need and stash the rest in the freezer.

INGREDIENTS

1 cup fresh or frozen strawberries
1 cup unsweetened apricot juice, chilled
½ cup plain low-fat yogurt
4 ice cubes (if using fresh fruit)

In a blender, combine strawberries, apricot juice, yogurt, and ice (if using) and blend until the mixture is smooth. Serve in 2 glasses.

PER SERVING: 130 calories, 1 g fat (0 g saturated fat), 4 g protein, 51 mg sodium, 27 g carbohydrates, 12.5 g sugars (0 g added sugar), 2 g fiber

---

Banana-Berry Blast Smoothie

VEGAN & HIGH FIBER!

Total time: 5 minutes
Makes: 2 servings

→ Get your morning off to a beautiful start with this tasty blend of fresh blueberries and your pick of raspberries or blackberries. In addition to being fiber stars, berries are loaded with skin-protecting antioxidants, including anthocyanins. And one serving of this smoothie powers you with all the collagen-stimulating vitamin C you need for the day!

INGREDIENTS

1 small ripe banana, sliced
¾ cup pineapple-orange juice
½ cup ice cubes
1 (6 ounce) container blueberries
1 (6 ounce) container raspberries or blackberries

1 teaspoon honey
1 teaspoon grated, peeled fresh ginger

In a blender, combine banana, pineapple-orange juice, ice, blueberries, raspberries or blackberries, honey, and ginger and blend until the mixture is smooth. Serve in 2 tall glasses.

PER SERVING: 196 calories, 1 g fat (0 g saturated fat), 3 g protein, 6 mg sodium, 48 g carbohydrates, 31 g sugars (3 g added sugar), 9 g fiber

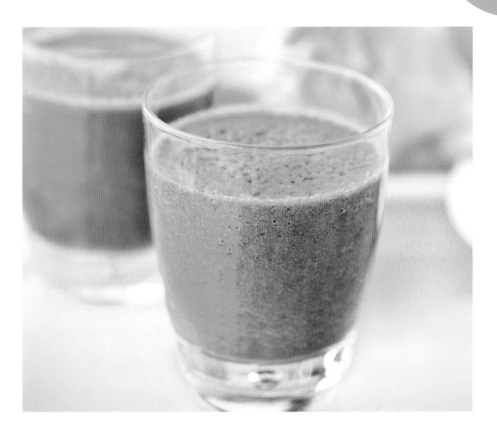

Lean, Mean & Green

Total time: 5 minutes
Makes: 2 servings

→ Tarragon brings a fresh note to this green blend. And bone broth adds protein (9 grams per serving!) plus collagen, which ups the elasticity and moisture in skin, according to some studies. Don't worry—your smoothie won't taste like chicken soup!

INGREDIENTS

1 (10 ounce) package frozen chopped spinach, broken up into chunks
2 medium Kirby cucumbers, peeled and sliced
1 cup apple juice
1 cup chicken bone broth
1 tablespoon fresh tarragon leaves

1. In a blender, combine spinach, cucumbers, apple juice, bone broth, and tarragon until smooth.

2. Strain mixture through a fine sieve into a large measuring cup; discard pulp. Serve in 2 tall glasses.

PER SERVING: 120 calories, 1 g fat (0 g saturated fat), 6 g protein, 120 mg sodium, 16 g carbohydrates, 13 g sugars (0 g added sugar), 2 g fiber

Green Papaya Cooler

Total time: 5 minutes
Makes: 1 serving

➜ Long known for its ability to hydrate, cucumber also contains caffeic acid and silica. Caffeic acid (also found in coffee) has anti-inflammatory benefits, and silica is a mineral that promotes the growth of healthy skin, nails, and cartilage.

INGREDIENTS
1 cup baby spinach
1 cup frozen papaya chunks
½ small cucumber, peeled and sliced
½ jalapeño, seeded
¼ cup refrigerated coconut milk

In a blender, combine spinach, papaya, cucumber, jalapeño, and coconut milk and blend until the mixture is smooth. Serve in a glass.

PER SERVING: 106 calories, 2 g fat (1 g saturated fat), 3 g protein, 68 mg sodium, 22 g carbohydrates, 14 g sugars (2 g added sugar), 5 g fiber

Tip To prep the jalapeño, halve the chile lengthwise, and then use a melon baller or the tip of a grapefruit spoon to remove the seeds. Be sure to wash your hands thoroughly after handling the pepper, and avoid touching your eyes!

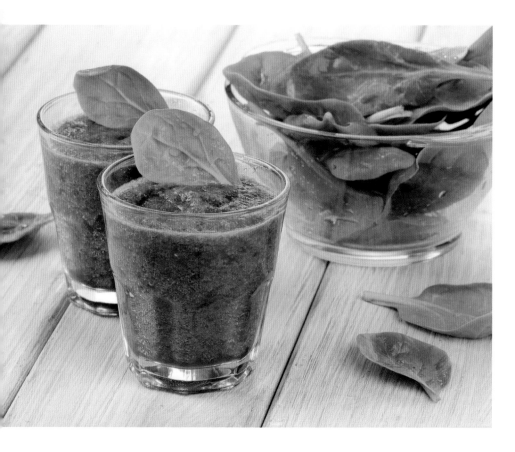

Tangy Mango Smoothie

Total time: 10 minutes
Makes: 1 serving

→ Mango is a skin-health hero! It's a good source of vitamin A, which helps draw water to the surface of the skin, helping to improve skin's texture and elasticity. The tropical fruit is also an excellent source of vitamin C (one serving contains 70 percent of the daily value), which plays an essential role in collagen synthesis and protects against UV-induced skin damage. And mango is also rich in copper, an essential mineral that plays a key role in making collagen.

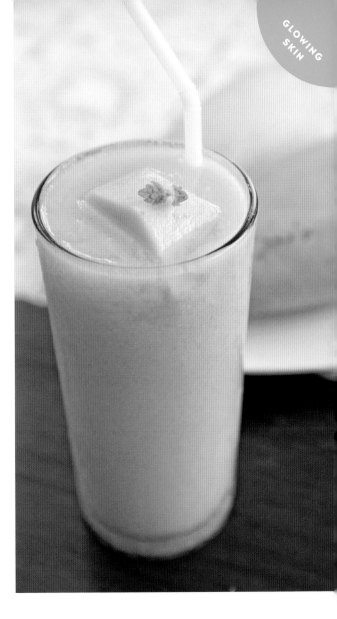

GLOWING SKIN

INGREDIENTS

1 medium ripe mango, cubed
¾ cup buttermilk
4 ice cubes
¼ teaspoon vanilla extract
Pinch of ground cardamom or cinnamon (optional)

In a blender, combine mango, buttermilk, ice, vanilla extract, and cardamom (if using) and blend until the mixture is smooth. Serve in a tall glass.

PER SERVING: 319 calories, 7 g fat (4 g saturated fat), 9 g protein, 196 mg sodium, 59 g carbohydrates, 54 g sugars (0 g added sugar), 5 g fiber

Tip No buttermilk? Make your own! Place 5 teaspoons lemon juice or white vinegar in a glass measuring cup, add enough low-fat (1 percent) milk to equal 5 cups, and stir. Let stand 5 minutes, then use in recipes.

Tropical Carrot Tango

Total time: 10 minutes
Makes: 2 servings

→ In this zesty drink, the much-loved veggie gets a vibrant tropical makeover with the addition of coconut milk, ginger, and pineapple. And the carrots deliver more than 100 percent of the recommended dietary allowance of skin-loving vitamin A. Add this sipper to your weekly skin-care regimen.

INGREDIENTS
1 cup refrigerated coconut milk
1 cup frozen pineapple chunks
¾ cup freshly grated, peeled carrot
¼ cup cold water
½-inch piece peeled, fresh ginger, sliced
1 teaspoon maple syrup

In a blender, combine coconut milk, pineapple, carrot, water, ginger, and maple syrup until smooth. Serve in 2 glasses.

PER SERVING: 106 calories, 3 g fat (3 g saturated fat), 1 g protein, 53 mg sodium, 21 g carbohydrates, 15 g sugars (5 g added sugar), 2 g fiber

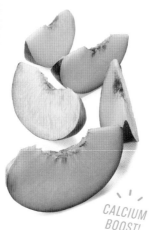

CALCIUM BOOST!

Tropical Peach Smoothie

Total time: 20 minutes
Makes: 2 servings

→ Fresh peaches, a good source of vitamins A and C, combine with supersweet mango, which is also loaded with vitamins A and C, for a skin-lifting tropical twist.

INGREDIENTS
1 pound peaches, sliced
1 cup frozen diced mango
½ cup unsweetened apple juice
½ cup plain whole-milk yogurt

In a blender, combine peaches, mango, apple juice, and yogurt and blend until the mixture is smooth. Serve in 2 glasses.

PER SERVING: 211 calories, 3 g fat (1 g saturated fat), 5 g protein, 31 mg sodium, 47 g carbohydrates, 40 g sugars (0 g added sugar), 5 g fiber

Black & Blueberry Blizzard

Total time: 5 minutes
Makes: 1 serving

→ This gorgeous blend is packed with phytochemicals. One in particular, the hesperidin in orange juice, may fight age spots by reducing the amount of melanin that our skin produces. Let's drink to that!

INGREDIENTS
½ cup buttermilk
½ cup orange juice, chilled
1 cup frozen blueberries
½ cup frozen blackberries
½ teaspoon honey

In a blender, combine buttermilk, orange juice, blueberries, blackberries, and honey and blend until the mixture is smooth. Serve in a tall glass.

PER SERVING: 270 calories, 6 g fat (2 g saturated fat), 6 g protein, 132 mg sodium, 52 g carbohydrates, 40 g sugars (3 g added sugar), 8 g fiber

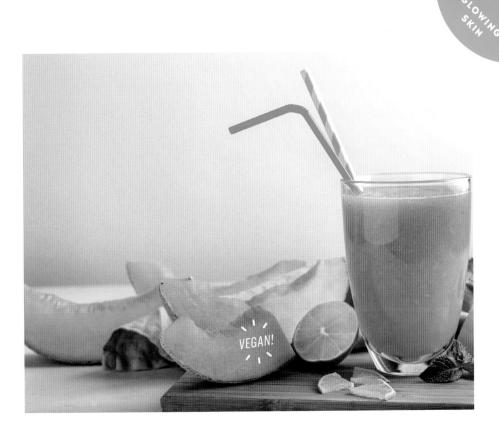

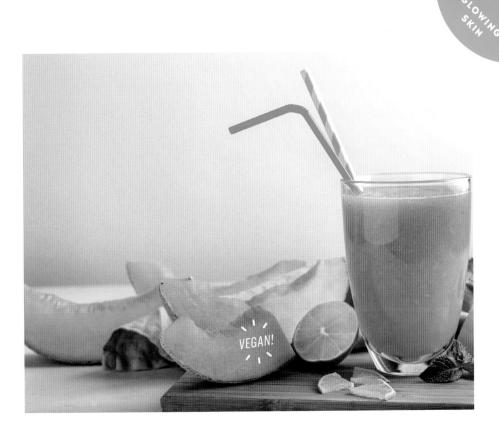

VEGAN!

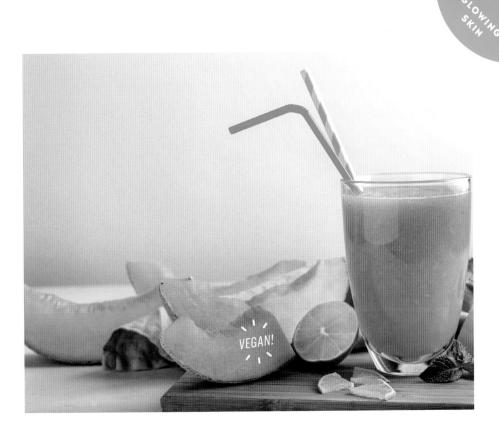

GLOWING SKIN

Cantaloupe-Lime Smoothie

Total time: 10 minutes
Makes: 1 serving

→ Both peaches and cantaloupe are loaded with skin-friendly beta-carotene. And cantaloupe is 90 percent water, so this smoothie helps plump and smooth your skin with every hydrating sip.

INGREDIENTS
1 lime
2 cups diced cantaloupe
⅓ cup diced peach
½ teaspoon honey
3 ice cubes

1. Prepare the lime (see tip), then grate ½ teaspoon zest and squeeze 2 tablespoons juice.

2. In a blender, combine lime zest and juice, cantaloupe, peach, honey, and ice; blend until the mixture is smooth. Serve in a tall glass.

PER SERVING: 147 calories, 1 g fat (0 g saturated fat), 3 g protein, 52 mg sodium, 37 g carbohydrates, 31 g sugars (3 g added sugar), 4 g fiber

Tip Get the most juice out of a lime by doing this first: Roll the lime on the counter, applying gentle pressure, then slice it in half crosswise and squeeze.

Chapter 3

Inflammation Fighters

f you feel as if you've seen the word *inflammation* in many health articles lately, you're right. Science has linked chronic inflammation with the diseases that kill the most people each year in the United States: heart disease, cancer, chronic lower respiratory disease, type 2 diabetes, and stroke. And inflammation is also at the root of other debilitating conditions, like inflammatory bowel disease (IBD), Alzheimer's, arthritis, and osteoporosis. Autoimmune diseases, like lupus and fibromyalgia, also have an inflammatory component.

Inflammation on its own is actually a good thing. When we injure ourselves, inflammation helps increase blood flow to the area to fight infection and speed healing. That type of inflammation is called acute, and it's a positive response. Chronic inflammation—the type that hangs around for months or years—is the kind we want to reduce. The good news is that several plant substances, known as phytochemicals, can help do just that. And choosing more fresh, whole foods instead of processed foods can go a long way toward dialing down your body's inflammatory response. Turn the page for delicious ways to start fighting inflammation, lowering your risk for disease, and feeling better today.

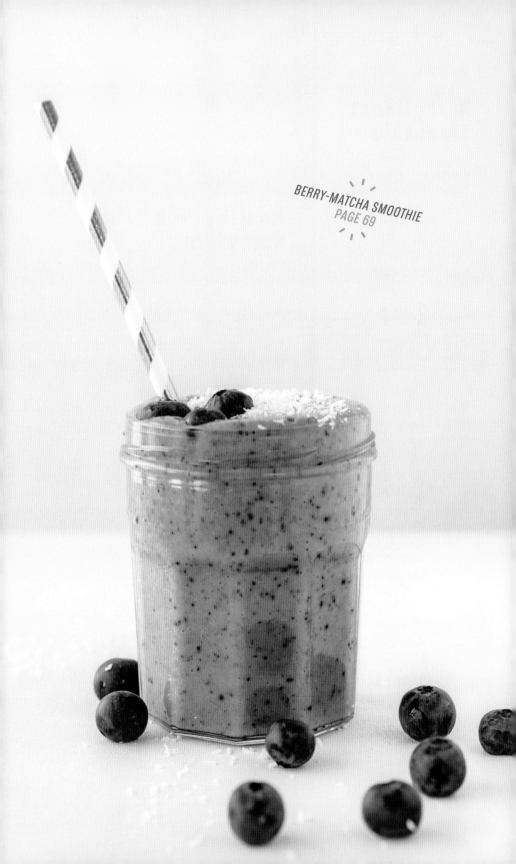

BERRY-MATCHA SMOOTHIE
PAGE 69

CALCIUM BOOST!

Berry Boost Smoothie

Total time: 5 minutes
Makes: 1 serving

➔ Pretty and sweet, strawberries also contain powerful anti-inflammatories. A study in the *British Journal of Nutrition* showed that strawberry extract helped fight the inflammatory response after a high-calorie meal. All the more reason to add them to your smoothies! This smoothie also delivers one-third of your recommended daily allowance of calcium.

INGREDIENTS
1 cup frozen strawberries
1 6-ounce container plain whole-milk yogurt
½ cup calcium-fortified orange juice
1 teaspoon honey

In a blender, combine strawberries, yogurt, orange juice, and honey and blend until the mixture is smooth. Serve in a tall glass.

PER SERVING: 236 calories, 6 g fat (4 g saturated fat), 7 g protein, 84 mg sodium, 41 g carbohydrates, 31 g sugars (6 g added sugar), 4 g fiber

Healthy Piña Colada Smoothie

Total time: 5 minutes
Makes: 4 servings

➔ Juicy pineapple delivers the taste of the tropics and also provides an anti-inflammatory benefit. Studies have shown that the bromelain enzyme in pineapple can alleviate the pain associated with osteoarthritis.

INGREDIENTS
1 ½ cups fresh or frozen pineapple chunks
1 ripe banana, sliced
14 ounce refrigerated, unsweetened coconut milk
1 6-ounce container vanilla whole-milk yogurt
½ cup ice cubes

In a blender, combine pineapple, banana, coconut milk, yogurt, and ice and blend until the mixture is smooth. Serve in 4 glasses.

PER SERVING:
133 calories, 4 g fat (3 g saturated fat), 3 g protein, 49 mg sodium, 24 g carbohydrates, 18 g sugars (5 g added sugar), 2 g fiber

Tip A fresh pineapple garnish adds tropical flair to this smoothie. Create your own by cutting a round from the middle of the pineapple and then slicing it into 4 wedges, leaving the skin on. Give the fruit a rinse before slicing into it.

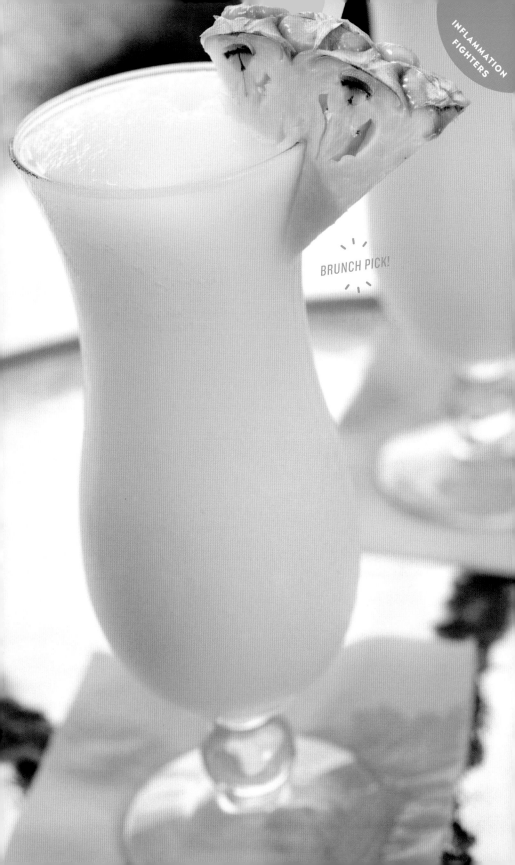

BRUNCH PICK!

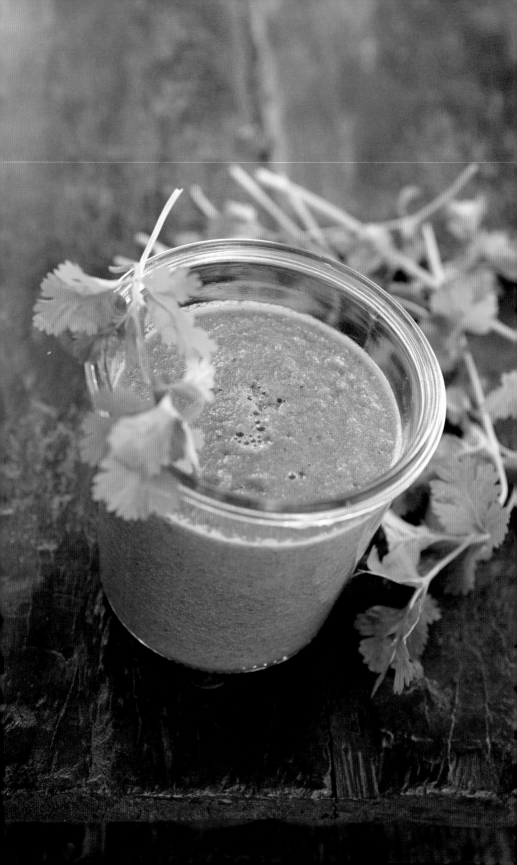

Ginger-Mango Smoothie

Total time: 10 minutes
Makes: 1 serving

→ Our citrusy smoothie features ginger, which may help soothe pain and calm an upset stomach. And the herb cilantro shows promise for use as an anti-inflammatory and antimicrobial. Cilantro can also help remove heavy metals from the body.

INGREDIENTS

½ cup spinach
½ cup frozen mango chunks
¼ cup Greek yogurt
3 tablespoons fresh orange juice
1 tablespoon fresh lemon juice
1-inch piece peeled fresh ginger
½ avocado
¼ cup water
Cilantro, for garnish (optional)

1. Blend spinach, mango, yogurt, orange juice, lemon juice, ginger, avocado, and water until smooth.

2. Serve in a tall glass. Garnish with cilantro, if desired.

PER SERVING: 236 calories, 11 g fat (1.5 g saturated fat), 9 g protein, 21 mg sodium, 31 g carbohydrates, 21 g sugars (0 g added sugar), 7 g fiber

Tip
Got leftover cilantro? Make flavor cubes! In a blender, combine 2 cups washed cilantro leaves and stems with ⅓ cup extra-virgin olive oil. Pour mixture into an ice cube tray and freeze until solid. Transfer cubes to an airtight plastic bag. This method works for any leafy herb. Add to dishes such as sauces or soups for a fresh flavor!

VEGAN & BREAKFAST TO GO!

Java Banana Smoothie

Total time: 5 minutes
Makes: 2 servings

→ Here's a frosty glass of joe with a bonus: Potassium-rich bananas help reduce blood pressure and risk for stroke. Plus, coffee contains polyphenols and other anti-inflammatory compounds that help combat inflammation.

INGREDIENTS

2 ripe bananas (preferably frozen), sliced in 1-inch rounds (see page 22)
¾ cup cold-brewed coffee (see page 124)
¾ cup unsweetened almond milk
1 cup ice cubes

In a blender, combine bananas, coffee, almond milk, and ice and blend well. Serve in 2 glasses.

PER SERVING: 293 calories, 2 g fat (0 g saturated fat), 2 g carbohydrates, 14 g sugars (0 g added sugar), 3 g fiber

Tip Hemp seeds contain high amounts of fatty acids, which can go rancid at room temperature. Store your hemp seeds (and other seeds) in the refrigerator or freezer to keep them fresh for up to a year.

Turmeric Twist

Total time: 5 minutes
Makes: 1 serving

→ Long used in Ayurvedic medicine, turmeric is a main component of curry powder and gives the powder its intense marigold color. Curcumin, the active ingredient in turmeric, has been found to help control pain from osteoarthritis as effectively as the painkiller ibuprofen does.

VEGAN!

INGREDIENTS

1 cup frozen mango chunks
½ cup refrigerated
   unsweetened coconut
   milk
¼ cup water
1 tablespoon hemp seeds
½ teaspoon ground ginger
½ teaspoon ground
   turmeric
Handful of ice
Honey, to taste (optional)

Blend mango, coconut milk, water, hemp seeds, ginger, turmeric, and ice until smooth. If you like, add honey to taste. Serve in a tall glass.

PER SERVING: 259 calories, 10 g fat (5 g saturated fat), 5 g protein, 39 mg sodium, 41 g carbohydrates, 31 g sugars (0 g added sugar), 5 g fiber

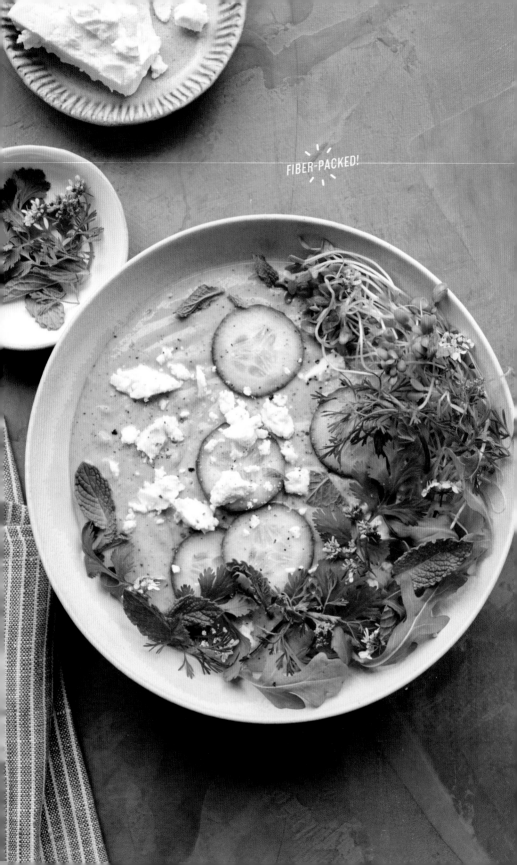

Herbal Healer Smoothie Bowl

Total time: 10 minutes
Makes: 2 servings

➜ Watch out, free radicals! The ingredients in this savory bowl may help squelch the damaging inflammatory molecules linked to cancer, diabetes, Alzheimer's, and more.

INGREDIENTS

FOR SMOOTHIE
1 cup low-fat buttermilk
½ cup fresh mint leaves
¼ cup cilantro
1 tablespoon lemon juice
1 teaspoon ground turmeric
1 cucumber, seeded and
    chopped
1 scallion
½ avocado
½ teaspoon black pepper
¼ teaspoon kosher salt

FOR TOPPING
½ cup baby arugula
½ cup sprouts
¼ cup crumbled feta
¼ cup fresh mint leaves
1 tablespoon cilantro sprigs
1 cucumber, sliced

1. Blend buttermilk, mint leaves, cilantro, lemon juice, turmeric, cucumber, scallion, avocado, pepper, and salt until smooth. Divide evenly between 2 bowls.

2. Top each bowl with ¼ cup arugula, ¼ cup sprouts, ⅛ cup feta, ⅛ cup mint leaves, ½ tablespoon cilantro sprigs, and half of the cucumber slices. Serve immediately.

PER SERVING: 221 calories, 10.5 g fat (4 g saturated fat), 13 g protein, 587 mg sodium, 23 g carbohydrates, 12 g sugars (0 g added sugar), 9 g fiber

---

Tip

Briny feta is a wonderful Mediterranean ingredient that can help punch up the flavor of salads, wraps, pasta, and more. It's much lower in calories per serving than most cheese. Store it in the brine that it comes in, or in olive oil in an airtight container to keep it fresh for weeks.

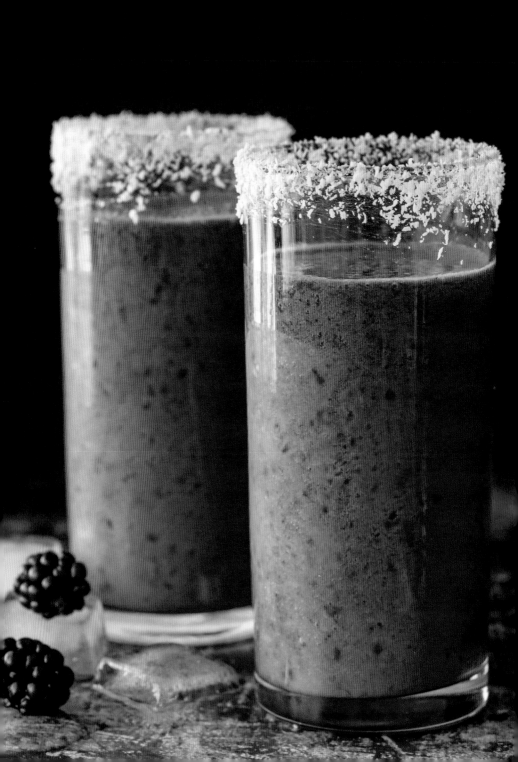

Four-Berry Belly Blast

Total time: 5 minutes
Makes: 2 servings

➜ If you're craving a frozen treat but watching your calories, try this healthy smoothie as a smart substitute for a sugary dessert. This slimming sipper is chock-full of four different berries and the health benefits that come with them. Anthocyanins, which give berries their bright colors, provide an anti-inflammatory hit that also looks great on your breakfast table.

INGREDIENTS

1 cup frozen mixed berries (blueberries, raspberries, blackberries, strawberries)
½ cup plain low-fat yogurt
½ cup orange juice
Shredded, unsweetened coconut (optional)

1. In a blender, combine berries, yogurt, and orange juice and blend until the mixture is smooth.

2. Serve in 2 glasses. Garnish with shredded coconut, if desired. If using, place the shredded coconut in a small bowl. Use a pastry brush or a paper towel to coat the inner and outer edge of 2 glasses with honey or agave syrup. Dip glasses in coconut to coat. Carefully fill glasses with smoothie and serve.

PER SERVING: 239 calories, 2 g fat (1 g saturated fat), 10 g protein, 88 mg sodium, 47 g carbohydrates, 31 g sugars (0 g added sugar), 7 g fiber

Tip Make an extra batch of this smoothie, pour into ice-pop molds, and freeze for six hours. You'll have a delicious, antioxidant-packed warm-weather treat!

Berry Good Smoothie

Total time: 10 minutes
Makes: 2 servings

→ Raspberries are not only sweet to eat but also tiny anti-inflammatory powerhouses. Ellagic acid, a polyphenol or plant compound rich with antioxidant activity, has been found to be particularly effective at fighting inflammation in the skin.

INGREDIENTS

1½ cups chopped
    strawberries
1 cup blueberries
½ cup raspberries
2 teaspoon honey
1 teaspoon fresh
    lemon juice
½ cup ice cubes

In a blender, combine strawberries, blueberries, raspberries, honey, lemon juice, and ice. Blend until the mixture is smooth. Serve in 2 tall glasses

PER SERVING: 120 calories,
1 g fat (0 g saturated fat),
2 g protein, 3 mg sodium,
30 g carbohydrates,
21 g sugars (6 g added sugar),
6 g fiber

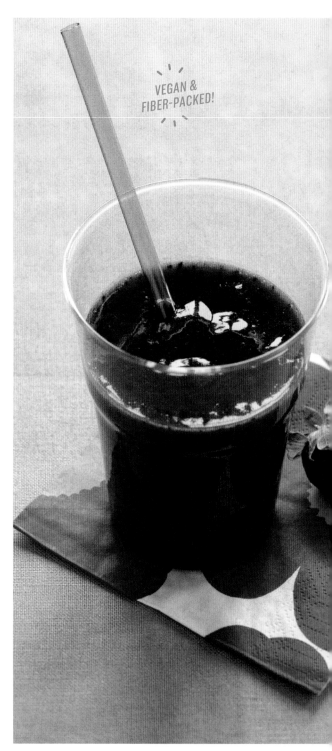

VEGAN &
FIBER-PACKED!

Berry-Matcha Smoothie

Total time: 10 minutes
Makes: 1 serving

➔ You already know that blueberries (both wild and regular) are good for you. Now research shows they may also help reduce age-related memory loss. One study found that older adults with memory loss who drank wild blueberry juice daily for 12 weeks had improved memory and reduced depressive symptoms. Experts believe the abundant anthocyanin antioxidants in berries may support brain cell communication, facilitate circulation, and protect neurons. Get your daily dose with this smoothie, which includes a cup of blueberries and other ingredients like spinach that are proven to ramp up brain health. See photo, page 57.

INGREDIENTS

1 cup fresh blueberries or frozen wild blueberries
¾ cup water
½ cup spinach
½ cup yogurt
¼ cup refrigerated unsweetened coconut milk
1 teaspoon matcha powder
½ teaspoon ground turmeric
Ice, as needed

1. Blend blueberries, water, spinach, yogurt, coconut milk, matcha, and turmeric until smooth.

2. Add ice, as needed, and blend again. Serve in a tall glass.

PER SERVING: 180 calories, 6 g fat (4 g saturated fat), 7 g protein, 70 mg sodium, 29 g carbohydrates, 21 g sugars (0 g added sugar), 4 g fiber

> *Tip*
> Matcha is expensive, so store yours properly for best results. Keep matcha powder in an opaque, airtight tin in the refrigerator to preserve the antioxidants and prevent the tea from breaking down and changing color. If stored properly, it will last several months.

PB&J Smoothie

Total time: 5 minutes
Makes: 2 servings

➜ Sweet and juicy, grapes are also an inflammation-fighting powerhouse. The polyphenols in grapes help stop chronic inflammation by reducing oxidative stress and preventing the activation of critical metabolic pathways that lead to inflammation. Grapes may play a role in protecting against decline in Alzheimer's-related areas of the brain.

INGREDIENTS

½ cup unsweetened hemp milk
3 tablespoons unsweetened natural peanut butter
2 tablespoons ground flaxseed
¾ cup red grapes, frozen
½ frozen banana

Blend hemp milk, peanut butter, ground flaxseed, grapes, and banana until smooth. Serve in 2 glasses.

PER SERVING: 279 calories, 17.5 g fat (2 g saturated fat), 8 g protein, 125 mg sodium, 25 g carbohydrates, 14 g sugars (0 g added sugar), 5 g fiber

---

Jump-Start Smoothie

Total time: 5 minutes
Makes: 2 servings

➜ If you're living with inflammation, it can be tough to get out of bed in the morning. Jump-start your day with this inflammation-fighting smoothie. Strawberries are packed with the phytochemical anthocyanin, as well as the B vitamin folate. The rheumatoid arthritis medication, methotrexate, lowers levels of folate, so there are multiple reasons to reach for this red berry.

INGREDIENTS

1 cup frozen strawberries
½ cup fresh blueberries
½ cup orange-tangerine juice blend, chilled
2 teaspoons chopped, peeled fresh ginger
¼ cup plain low-fat yogurt
2 ice cubes

In a blender, combine strawberries, blueberries, orange-tangerine juice, ginger, yogurt, and ice. Blend until the mixture is smooth. Serve in 2 tall glasses.

PER SERVING: 96 calories, 1 g fat (0 g saturated fat), 3 g protein, 24 mg sodium, 21 g carbohydrates, 15 g sugars (0 g added sugar), 2 g fiber

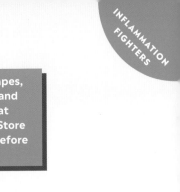

Tip If you see a cloudy coating on your grapes, that's a good thing. It's called bloom, and it's a naturally occurring substance that protects grapes from moisture loss and decay. Store your grapes in the fridge and wash them right before using to keep them at their freshest.

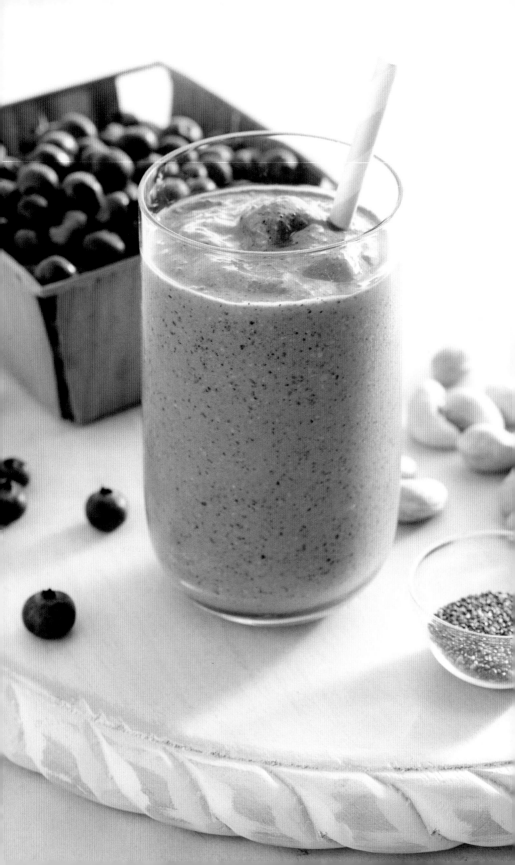

Blueberry-Cashew Bliss

Total time: 5 minutes
Makes: 2 servings

➔ Bliss out! The probiotics in yogurt have been shown to enhance mood. The hemp and chia both supply omega-3 and -6 fatty acids, and the hemp also offers up stearidonic (SDA) and gamma linolenic acids (GLA), which all deliver an anti-inflammatory benefit. Cashews also provide satisfying, healthy fats in this creamy drink.

INGREDIENTS

½ cup unsweetened hemp milk
½ cup plain Greek yogurt
1 tablespoon hulled hemp seeds
1 tablespoon chia seeds
1 cup frozen blueberries
½ frozen banana
¼ cup raw cashews
½ cup ice

Blend hemp milk, yogurt, hemp seeds, chia seeds, blueberries, banana, cashews, and ice until smooth. Serve in 2 glasses.

PER SERVING: 261 calories, 14.5 g fat (3 g saturated fat), 11 g protein, 55 mg sodium, 25 g carbohydrates, 13 g sugars (0 g added sugar), 5g fiber

---

VEGAN & MEAL-PREP IDEA!

Green Piña Colada

Total time: 5 minutes
Makes: 2 servings

➔ This tropical smoothie has the added benefit of kaempferol, a flavonoid found in spinach and other vegetables that shows both an anti-inflammatory and antimicrobial benefit in preliminary studies. Prep this smoothie in advance and blend it up whenever you need a healing start to the day.

INGREDIENTS
FREEZE:
1 cup pineapple chunks
1 banana, sliced
2 cups baby spinach

ADD:
1 cup refrigerated coconut milk

1. Place pineapple, banana, and spinach in a zip-top plastic bag or freezer-safe jar. Freeze overnight or longer.

2. When ready to prepare, add coconut milk to a blender, then add frozen ingredients and blend until smooth.

3. Pour into 2 tall glasses and serve immediately.

PER SERVING: 185 calories, 7.5 g fat (7 g saturated fat), 4 g protein, 55 mg sodium, 28 g carbohydrates, 17 g sugars (3 g added sugar), 4 g fiber

Tip The easiest way to slice up a pineapple is to place it on its side on a cutting board and remove the top and bottom of the fruit. Stand the pineapple up and use a sharp knife to slice off the brown rind. Cut the fruit in half and remove the tough inner core. Cut the remaining fruit into chunks.

Get-Ahead Gingerbread Smoothie

Total time: 10 minutes
Makes: 1 serving

→ The warm spices in gingerbread help turn down inflammation. A study in the *International Journal of Preventive Medicine* found that both ginger and cinnamon contribute to the alleviation of soreness.

INGREDIENTS

7 ounces 2 percent Greek yogurt
1 cup ice cubes
¼ cup frozen sliced banana
2 tablespoons almond butter
1 teaspoon molasses
1 teaspoon freshly grated ginger
¼ teaspoon ground cinnamon
⅛ teaspoon ground nutmeg
⅛ teaspoon ground cardamom

Blend yogurt, ice, banana, almond butter, molasses, ginger, cinnamon, nutmeg, and cardamom until smooth. Serve in a tall glass.

PER SERVING: 400 calories, 22 g fat (4 g saturated fat), 27 g protein, 73 mg sodium, 29 g carbohydrates, 18 g sugars (5 g added sugar), 5 g fiber

POWER UP!

Add extra nutrients to your daily smoothie with these healthy add-ins:

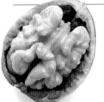

Protein: peanut, almond, or cashew butter; silken tofu; whey, pea, hemp, or other protein powder (turn to page 13 for more on picking the protein powder that's right for you).

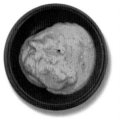

Omega-3 fats: chia seeds, ground flaxseed, hemp seeds, walnuts

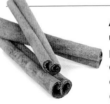

Antioxidants: unsweetened cocoa powder, turmeric, cinnamon, nutmeg, cardamom, wheat germ, matcha powder, bee pollen, fresh or ground ginger, fresh herbs

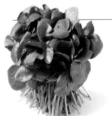

Iron: baby spinach, kale, watercress, parsley

VEGAN & VITAMIN C STAR!

Healthy High C Smoothie

Total time: 10 minutes
Makes: 2 servings

→ Studies have shown that the antioxidant vitamin C helps your body kick out damaging free radicals, which leads to less inflammation. The trio of kale, kiwi, and OJ in this healthy shake add up to more than 100 percent of your RDA for vitamin C.

INGREDIENTS
1 cup chopped kale leaves, stems and ribs removed and discarded
2 large kiwifruits, peeled and chopped
½ cup fresh orange juice
½ cup cilantro sprigs
1 stalk celery, chopped
¼ cup ice cubes

In a blender, combine kale, kiwifruits, orange juice, cilantro, celery, and ice. Blend until the mixture is smooth. Serve in 2 tall glasses.

PER SERVING: 180 calories, 1 g fat (0 g saturated fat), 2 g protein, 24 mg sodium, 21 g carbohydrates, 13 sugars (0 g added sugar), 3 g fiber

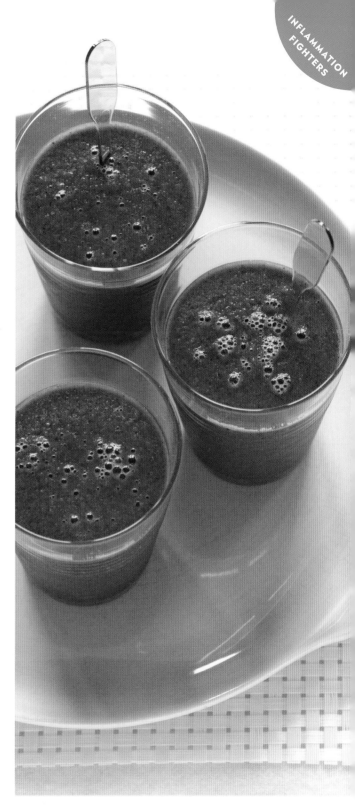

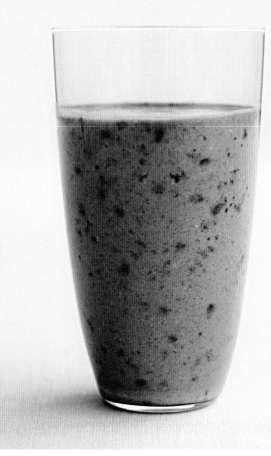

Pomegranate-Berry

Total time: 5 minutes
Makes: 1 serving

➜ Love the tangy-sweet flavor of pomegranate juice? It's time to raise a glass. Research shows that polyphenol-rich pomegranate juice can help fight inflammation related to diseases such as rheumatoid arthritis, inflammatory bowel disease, and metabolic and cardiovascular disorders.

Tip   **Mix it up!** Frozen mixed berries typically include strawberries, blueberries, raspberries, and blackberries, but that doesn't mean you can't create your own blend. Try a 1-cup mix of frozen dark sweet cherries, raspberries, and wild blueberries.

INGREDIENTS
½ cup pomegranate juice, chilled
½ cup vanilla low-fat yogurt
1 cup frozen mixed berries

In a blender, combine pomegranate juice, yogurt, and berries and blend until the mixture is smooth. Serve in a tall glass.

PER SERVING: 250 calories, 2 g fat (1 g saturated fat), 6 g protein, 110 mg sodium, 52 g carbohydrates, 44 g sugars (8 g added sugar), 5 g fiber

VEGAN!

Banana, Berry, and Pineapple Smoothie

Total time: 10 minutes
Makes: 1 serving

→ Packed with the antioxidant flavonoid anthocyanin, blackberries may aid in reducing oxidative stress, turning down inflammation in the body, and supporting immune system function.

INGREDIENTS
1 small banana
¾ cup unsweetened pineapple juice
½ cup ice cubes
1 cup blueberries
1 cup blackberries
1 teaspoon honey
1 teaspoon grated, peeled fresh ginger

In a blender, combine banana, pineapple juice, ice, blueberries, blackberries, honey, and ginger and blend until the mixture is smooth. Serve in a tall glass.

PER SERVING: 358 calories, 2 g fat (0 g saturated fat), 5 g protein, 8 mg sodium, 89 g carbohydrates, 58 sugars (6 g added sugar), 14 g fiber

VEGAN!

Spicy Green Smoothie

Total time: 10 minutes
Makes: 1 serving

→ Jalapeño pepper gives this vegan smoothie its zesty kick (and may also help combat inflammation). Kale is rich in vitamin K, a fat-soluble vitamin that plays a key role in blood clotting and bone health. Vitamin K also lowers inflammatory markers in the body and may contribute to the fight against heart disease and osteoporosis. The heart-healthy fats in avocado help ensure you absorb the vitamin K.

INGREDIENTS
1 ¼ cups water
½ celery stalk, chopped
½ cucumber, sliced
¼ avocado, pitted and peeled
2 kale leaves, stems and ribs removed and discarded
1 tablespoon chopped fresh cilantro
1 tablespoon fresh lemon juice
¼ jalapeño, with seeds

In a blender, combine water, celery, cucumber, avocado, kale, cilantro, lemon juice, and jalapeño and blend until the mixture is smooth. Serve in a tall glass.

PER SERVING: 114 calories, 8 g fat (1 g saturated fat), 3 g protein, 23 mg sodium, 11 g carbohydrates, 4 g sugars (0 g added sugar), 6 g fiber

Tip If you prefer your smoothie less spicy, remove the vein and seeds from the jalapeño—they're the hottest parts. And don't touch your eyes after slicing into it!

77

Powered-Up Purple Smoothie

Total time: 10 minutes
Makes: 1 serving

➜ We can barely keep track of all the superfoods in this delicious smoothie. Kale, blueberries, yogurt, and flaxseeds—wow! Flaxseeds are often touted for their ability to lower cholesterol, but research shows they also help reduce inflammation that leads to cardiovascular disease.

INGREDIENTS

½ cup unsweetened almond milk
½ cup nonfat Greek yogurt
⅔ cup kale
1 cup blueberries
1 teaspoon ground flaxseed
1 teaspoon honey

In a blender, combine almond milk, yogurt, kale, blueberries, ground flaxseed, and honey. Blend until the mixture is smooth. Serve in a tall glass.

PER SERVING: 210 calories, 4 g fat (0 g saturated fat), 14 g protein, 137 mg sodium, 34 g carbohydrates, 24 g sugars (6 g added sugar), 5 g fiber

> *Tip* You can buy ground flaxseed, but grinding it yourself ensures it's at its optimal freshness. Grind flaxseeds in a blender or a clean coffee grinder to release their healthy nutrients. If using a blender, be sure to grind the flaxseeds before adding other smoothie ingredients.

Green Light

Total time: 5 minutes
Makes: 1 serving

➜ Green means go for this blender juice! Kale, grapes, and ginger slip a triple threat of anti-inflammatory power into one tasty glass.

INGREDIENTS

4 kale leaves, stems and ribs removed and discarded
1 cup coconut water
1 cup seedless green grapes
1 small (½ inch) piece peeled fresh ginger, sliced

1. In a blender, combine kale, coconut water, grapes, and ginger and blend until the mixture is smooth.

2. Strain the smoothie through a fine sieve into a large measuring cup; discard the pulp.

3. Serve in a tall glass.

PER SERVING: 155 calories, 0 g fat (0 g saturated fat), 1 g protein, 50 mg sodium, 37 g carbohydrates, 32 g sugars (0 g added sugar), 1 g fiber

To peel ginger, use a vegetable peeler or the edge of a teaspoon to scrape away the thin skin. Be careful to remove only the very top layer of skin, because the flesh directly beneath is the youngest and most delicate.

YOUR INFLAMMATION-FIGHTING SHOPPING LIST

Before we stock your shelves, let's talk about what shouldn't be on them. Added sugars, refined carbohydrates, and saturated and trans fats all create inflammation. And since inflammation is linked to high blood pressure, it also makes sense to limit sodium to the recommended 2,300 milligrams per day. Keep the following foods on rotation in your smoothies and for snacks.

GRAPES

These super snackers are also rich in anti-inflammatories. Their mix of flavonoids and resveratrol combine to fight free radicals and inflammation. Resveratrol shows promise in combating the inflammatory effects of Parkinson's disease, Alzheimer's, and other age-related illnesses. Harness the power of grapes in these recipes: PB&J Smoothie (page 70), Green Light (page 78), Green Team Smoothie (page 96), and Great Grape Smoothie (page 100).

CHERRIES

Cherries offer a wealth of inflammation-busting power in their small scarlet package. Studies have found that cherries, both sweet and tart, help prevent or decrease oxidative stress and inflammation in the body. Both sweet and tart cherry varieties are rich in polyphenols, including anthocyanins. Add cherries to your anti-inflammatory diet with these delicious smoothies: Workout Recovery Smoothie (page 110) and Cherry-Almond Smoothie (page 119).

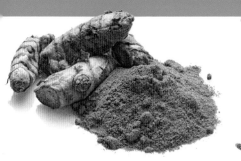

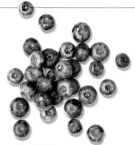

TURMERIC

This spice is a component of curry powder and serves up a bevy of anti-inflammatory benefits. The active ingredient in turmeric, curcumin, has been shown to help with symptoms of irritable bowel syndrome (IBS), stomach ulcers, and Crohn's disease. It can also help with the pain of post-operative inflammation and rheumatoid arthritis. Unlock the pain-fighting power of turmeric with these recipes: Turmeric Twist (page 63), Herbal Healer Smoothie Bowl (page 65), and Berry-Matcha Smoothie (page 69).

CHIA SEEDS

Small and mighty, chia seeds were prized by the Aztecs and Mayans for the long-lasting energy they provide. The seeds contain alpha-linolenic acid, a type of plant-based omega-3 fatty acid that has anti-inflammatory benefits. Power up with chia in these recipes: Blueberry-Cashew Bliss Smoothie (page 73), Pineapple-Citrus Smoothie Bowl (page 85), Banana-Berry Smoothie Bowl (page 23), and Sun Shake (page 46).

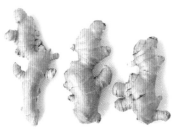

GINGER

The zing that ginger gives to food is delicious, but this ancient healing ingredient also has a ton of inflammation-fighting power. In studies, ginger has been linked to relieving menstrual pain, pain from migraines, and pain from rheumatoid arthritis and osteoarthritis. Reach for these smoothies to benefit from ginger's healing powers: Ginger-Mango Smoothie (page 61), Turmeric Twist (page 63), Get-Ahead Gingerbread Smoothie (page 74), Jump-Start Smoothie (page 70), Banana, Berry, and Pineapple Smoothie (page 77), and Green Light (page 78).

BLUEBERRIES AND WILD BLUEBERRIES

These tart-sweet gems are tiny but formidable inflammation fighters. Blueberries contain high amounts of anthocyanins, a type of antioxidant that counters inflammation and may help reduce the risk for heart disease and cancer. These berries show promise as an aid in reducing age-related cognitive decline, thanks to their high polyphenol content. Sip on these smoothies to reap blueberries' benefits: Four-Berry Belly Blast (page 67), Berry-Matcha Smoothie (page 69), Blueberry-Cashew Bliss Smoothie (page 73), Berry Good Smoothie (page 68), Jump-Start Smoothie (page 70), and Pomegranate-Berry Smoothie (page 76).

Chapter 4

Healthy Heart

No other muscle in the body is the subject of poems and movie titles (and it's not like people are texting calf muscle emojis to each other). That's probably because without a healthy, beating heart, we cease to exist. And yet heart disease continues to be the number one disease affecting women and men in the United States.

It's true that nearly everything we do affects our heart. The activity we do, the air we breathe, and the food and drink we consume all have the ability to enhance or diminish the health of this fist-size organ. All the recipes collected in this chapter feature ingredients that help make our hearts beat more strongly and our blood pump more freely, and that's reason enough to share these recipes with the ones you love.

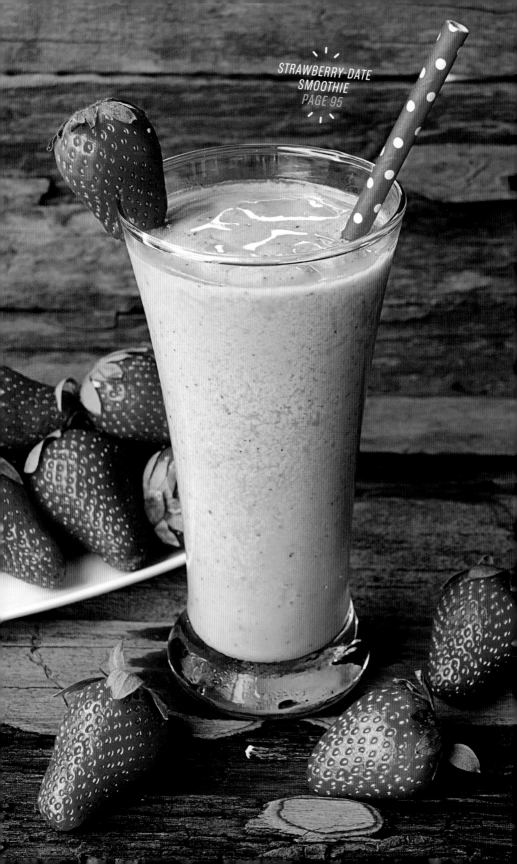

STRAWBERRY-DATE
SMOOTHIE
PAGE 95

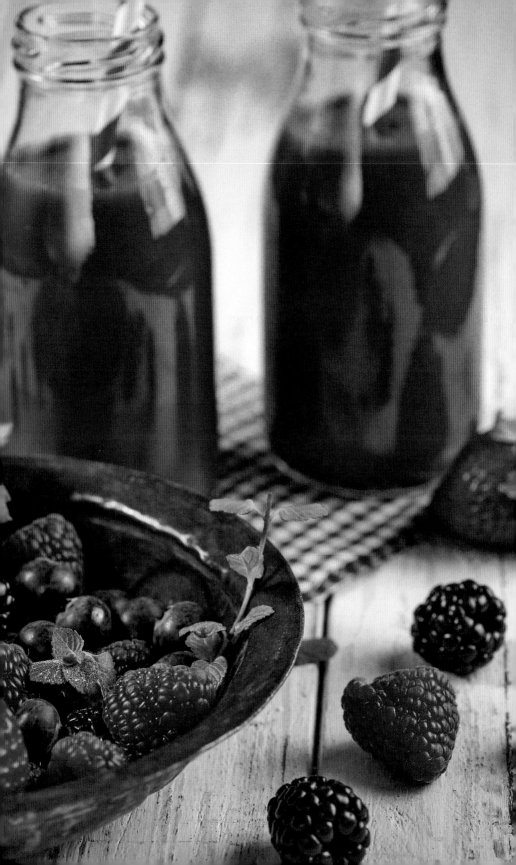

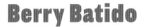
Berry Batido

Total time: 5 minutes
Makes: 1 serving

→ Batidos (also known as licuados) are the Latin American version of fruit smoothies. We added walnuts to this fiber-packed recipe for a subtle crunch and for their cardio-protective benefits. A recent Penn State study found that a diet low in saturated fats and containing walnuts helps lower central blood pressure, the type that is exerted on vital organs like the heart.

INGREDIENTS

1 cup frozen strawberries
1 cup frozen blueberries or blackberries
1 cup raspberries
1 cup goji berries (optional)
1 ripe banana, sliced
1 tablespoon walnuts, chopped

In a blender, combine strawberries, blueberries, raspberries, goji berries (if using), banana, and walnuts and blend until the mixture is smooth. Serve in a tall glass.

PER SERVING: 545 calories, 7 g fat (1 g saturated fat), 6 g protein, 7 mg sodium, 78 g carbohydrates, 42 g sugars (0 g added sugar), 18 g fiber

VEGAN!

Pineapple-Citrus Smoothie

Total time: 5 minutes
Makes: 1 serving

→ Sunshine in a glass! And it's a nutritional knockout to boot. The combined potassium in the orange juice, carrot juice, pineapple, and banana add up to a whopping 1,185 milligrams, which is nearly half the daily potassium requirement for women. Potassium plays a key role in heart health (see page 106 for more on potassium), and low levels of this essential nutrient are linked to high blood pressure, heart disease, and stroke.

INGREDIENTS

¾ cup orange juice, chilled
¾ cup carrot juice, chilled
1 cup frozen pineapple chunks
½ frozen banana, sliced

In a blender, combine orange juice, carrot juice, pineapple, and banana and blend until the mixture is smooth and frothy. Serve in a tall glass.

PER SERVING: 297 calories, 0 g fat (0 g saturated fat), 5 g protein, 115 mg sodium, 73 g carbohydrates, 34 g sugars (0 g added sugar), 6 g fiber

Tip **The more sodium there is in your diet, the more potassium you need. If you know you're going to have a high-sodium day (Bloody Marys with brunch or pizza night), be sure to start it off with a high-potassium smoothie like this one.**

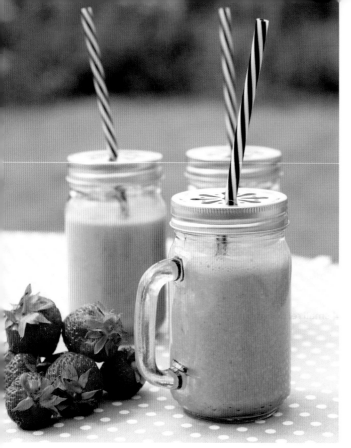

Strawberries & Cream Smoothie

Total time: 5 minutes
Makes: 2 servings

→ Deliciously fragrant and sweet, strawberries are also your heart's best friend. A study at Oklahoma State University on the effects of strawberries on heart disease risk factors revealed that participants who consumed the most freeze-dried berries over 12 weeks had the greatest decrease in both total and LDL (bad) cholesterol.

INGREDIENTS
1 pound strawberries, hulled
1 cup frozen peach slices
¼ cup vanilla low-fat yogurt
¼ cup unsweetened almond milk
1 teaspoon honey

In a blender, combine strawberries, peach slices, yogurt, almond milk, and honey and blend until the mixture is smooth. Serve in 2 glasses.

PER SERVING: 135 calories, 1.5 g fat (0 g saturated fat), 4 g protein, 45 mg sodium, 31 g carbohydrates, 24 g sugars (5 g added sugar), 5 g fiber

Tip
When strawberries are in season, buy an extra one-pound container for another batch of these creamy smoothies later in the week. Arrange the berries (without washing or stemming) on a paper towel-lined tray, cover with plastic wrap, and refrigerate. Before using, wash under cool water and then remove the stems. Washing right before use will prevent the berries from turning moldy from excess moisture.

Mighty Veggie Smoothie

Total time: 5 minutes
Makes: 2 servings

→ Not a fan of beets? This tasty smoothie will change your mind. Plus, beets are one of the richest sources of nitrates, which aid blood flow, reduce blood pressure, and support heart health. And studies have shown that they help improve exercise ability in patients with heart failure. Garnish this beauty with fresh mint and dark chocolate shavings for an extra flavor boost.

INGREDIENTS

4 small refrigerated cooked beets, sliced in 1-inch rounds
¾ cup shredded carrots
1 cup orange juice
2 frozen ripe bananas, sliced
1 tablespoon ground flaxseed

In a blender, combine beets, carrots, orange juice, bananas, and flaxseed and blend until the mixture is smooth. Serve in 2 glasses.

PER SERVING: 228 calories, 2 g fat (0 g saturated fat), 4 g protein, 48 mg sodium, 51 g carbohydrates, 32 g sugars (0 g added sugar), 7 g fiber

VEGAN!

Beet-Citrus Blast

Total time: 5 minutes
Makes: 1 serving

→ Like the Mighty Veggie Smoothie (page 87), this bright-red drink also delivers the heart-smart benefits of beets. Plus, it contains navel oranges, which are rich in potassium, another potent blood vessel relaxer. Tiny hemp seeds contain an ideal ratio of omega-6 to omega-3 fatty acids for reducing heart disease risks, as well as plant chemicals thought to lower blood pressure.

INGREDIENTS

1 beet, peeled and chopped
1 navel orange, peeled
2 tablespoons hemp seeds
1-inch piece fresh ginger,
    peeled and grated
Handful of ice

In a blender, combine beet, orange, hemp seeds, ginger, and ice and blend until the mixture is smooth. Serve in a tall glass.

PER SERVING: 219 calories, 8.5 g fat (0.5 g saturated fat), 9 g protein, 66 mg sodium, 29 g carbohydrates, 18 g sugars (0 g added sugar), 5 g fiber

VEGAN!

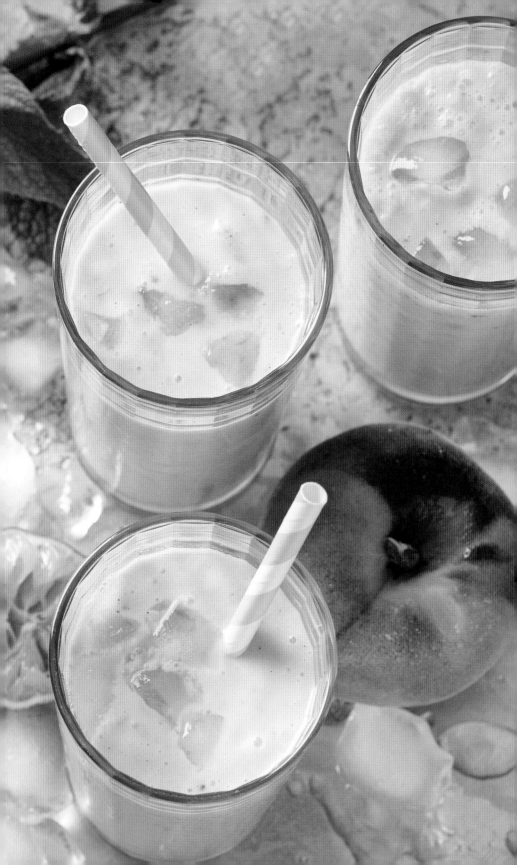

Stone Fruit Smoothie

Total time: 5 minutes
Makes: 2 servings

→ This sweet smoothie delivers a full serving of fruit! What's more, stone fruit, including the ones featured in this recipe, show promise in reducing heart disease risk by lowering inflammation in the body. Fresh stone fruit is at its peak in late spring and into summer, but you can use frozen during the rest of the year. Delicate white tea provides an added helping of antioxidants.

INGREDIENTS

1 plum, pitted and quartered
1 nectarine, pitted and quartered
1 peach, pitted and quartered
½ cup brewed white tea, chilled
½ cup ice cubes
2 tablespoons fresh lime juice
1 teaspoon honey
⅛ teaspoon ground cardamom (optional)

In a blender, combine plum, nectarine, peach, white tea, ice, lime juice, honey, and cardamom (if using) and blend until the mixture is smooth. Serve in 2 glasses.

PER SERVING: 90 calories, 0 g fat (0 g saturated fat), 2 g protein, 1 mg sodium, 23 g carbohydrates, 18 g sugars (3 g added sugar), 3 g fiber

Tip **You can substitute black, green, or herbal tea for the white tea.**

Double Orange Smoothie

Total time: 10 minutes
Makes: 2 servings

→ A double dose of orange means a double dose of powerful nutrients! Hesperidin, a flavonoid found in oranges and grapefruits, helps reduce inflammation and supports healthy blood vessels. And don't worry about juicing fresh oranges. Commercially squeezed oranges contain higher amounts of hesperidin.

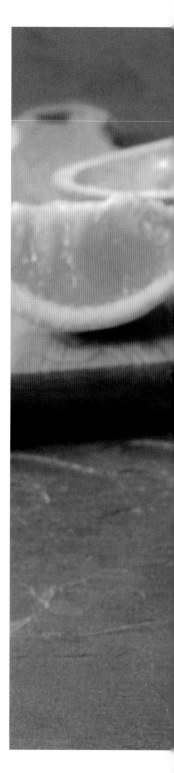

INGREDIENTS

1 navel or blood orange, peeled
1 cup vanilla low-fat yogurt
1 cup ice cubes
½ cup orange juice
2 teaspoons honey

1. Section orange; transfer sections to a small freezer-safe container. Cover and freeze until sections are very cold, about 20 minutes.
2. In a blender, combine yogurt, ice, orange juice, honey, and frozen orange sections and blend until smooth. Serve in 2 glasses.

PER SERVING:

188 calories, 2 g fat
(1 g saturated fat),
7 g protein, 82 mg sodium,
37 g carbohydrates,
34 sugars (14 g added sugar),
2 g fiber

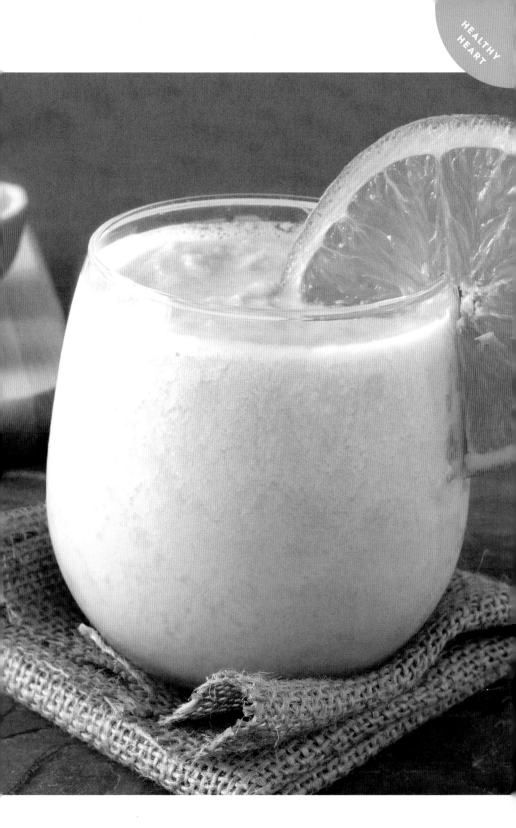

Healthy Banana Milkshake

Total time: 5 minutes
Makes: 2 servings

➜ A banana provides more than great taste in your smoothie. For a measly 100 calories, a medium-size fruit delivers about 450 milligrams of potassium. And half of a creamy avocado contributes 975 milligrams, making this smoothie super heart-friendly. According to the National Heart, Lung, and Blood Institute of the National Institutes of Health, a high intake of this mineral may stave off high blood pressure and improve blood pressure control in people who already have hypertension.

INGREDIENTS

½ avocado, pitted and peeled, plus more for garnish, optional
1 frozen ripe banana, sliced
1 cup unsweetened almond milk
1 teaspoon almond butter
1 teaspoon vanilla extract

In a blender, combine avocado, banana, almond milk, almond butter, and vanilla extract and blend until the mixture is smooth. Pour into two tall glasses, garnish with avocado slices, if using, and serve.

PER SERVING: 175 calories, 11 g fat (1 g saturated fat), 3 g protein, 94 mg sodium, 20 g carbohydrates, 8 g sugars (0 g added sugar), 6 g fiber

VEGAN!

VEGAN!

Strawberry-Date Smoothie

Total time: 5 minutes
Makes: 2 servings

➜ Dates are nutrient-dense and naturally supersweet, which means you don't have to add any sweetener when you include them in smoothies and other recipes. And while they are rich in natural sugars, dates are beneficial for diabetics. One study showed that when healthy participants ate 100 grams of dates daily for one month, their serum triglycerides decreased and blood glucose did not increase. Pair that with the heart benefits of strawberries and you get one health-revving glass.

INGREDIENTS

1 cup unsweetened almond milk
8 ice cubes
6 frozen strawberries
3 pitted dates
¼ teaspoon vanilla extract
Pinch of salt

In a blender, combine almond milk, ice, strawberries, dates, vanilla extract, and salt and blend until the mixture is smooth. Pour into two tall glasses and serve.

PER SERVING:

156 calories, 2 g fat (0 g saturated fat), 1 g protein, 149 mg sodium, 12 g carbohydrates, 8 sugars (0 g added sugar), 2 g fiber

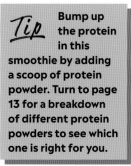

Tip **Bump up the protein in this smoothie by adding a scoop of protein powder. Turn to page 13 for a breakdown of different protein powders to see which one is right for you.**

Cocoa-Almond Smoothie

Total time: 5 minutes
Makes: 2 servings

➜ What's so brilliant about cocoa beyond its rich flavor? It's a good source of iron, magnesium, and zinc and clocks in at almost 2 grams of fiber per tablespoon. But most important, cocoa delivers flavanols, which help lower blood pressure, improve blood flow to the brain and heart, and make platelets (the component in blood that forms clots) less sticky, which allows blood to move more freely throughout the body.

INGREDIENTS
2 ripe bananas (preferably frozen), sliced into 1-inch rounds (see page 22 for tips on freezing bananas)
3 pitted dates
2 tablespoons unsweetened cocoa powder
¾ cup unsweetened almond milk
2 tablespoons almond butter
1 cup ice cubes
Dark chocolate shavings, optional

In a blender, combine bananas, dates, cocoa, almond milk, almond butter, and ice and blend until the mixture is smooth. Pour into 2 glasses or jars, add chocolate shavings on top, if using, and serve.

PER SERVING: 260 calories, 11 g fat (1 g saturated fat), 6 g protein, 71 mg sodium, 42 g carbohydrates, 22 sugars (0 g added sugar), 28 g fiber

---

Green Team Smoothie

Total time: 5 minutes
Makes: 2 servings

➜ Sweet, juicy, and fun to eat, grapes also offer up a host of health benefits. Human studies show that eating a variety of grapes may help keep your heart healthy by relaxing blood vessels, which maintains optimal blood flow and function.

INGREDIENTS
1 ½ cups unsweetened almond milk
1 medium Kirby cucumber, peeled and sliced into 1-inch rounds
1 cup green seedless grapes (preferably frozen)
2 medium stalks celery, peeled and sliced
1 teaspoon honey

In a blender, combine almond milk, cucumber, grapes, celery, and honey and blend until the mixture is smooth. Serve in 2 tall glasses.

PER SERVING: 103 calories, 2.5 g fat (0 g saturated fat), 2 g protein, 169 mg sodium, 20 g carbohydrates, 16 g sugars (3 g added sugar), 2 g fiber

Tip Freeze extra grapes to snack on! They make a super-hydrating post-workout snack. Simply rinse grapes and drain well. Place grape clusters on a cookie sheet and put in the freezer. Freeze for 2 hours and enjoy!

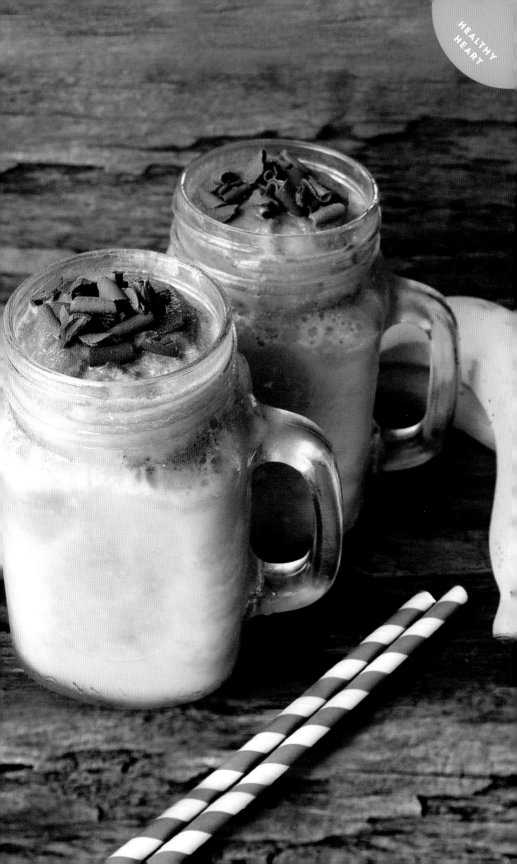

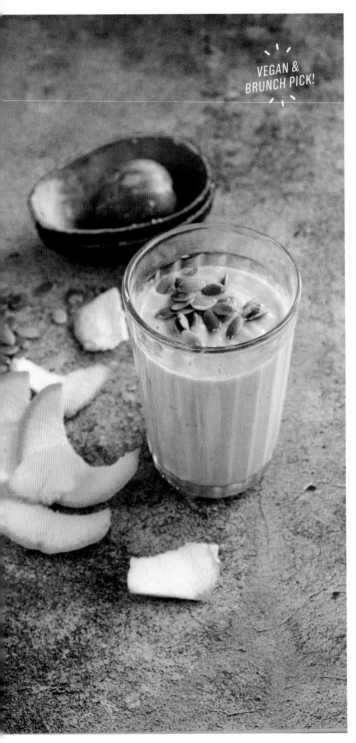

Berry, Orange & Avocado Smoothie

Total time: 10 minutes
Makes: 4 servings

→ This luscious smoothie gets a major green boost from tender baby spinach. And together, the ingredients offer a dose of potassium that adds up to 734 milligrams per serving, which is nearly 30 percent of your adequate intake (AI) for the day. Bottoms up!

INGREDIENTS

1 avocado, pitted and
   peeled
2 ½ cups orange juice
2 cups frozen mixed berries
2 cups packed baby spinach
2 cups ice cubes

In a blender, combine avocado, orange juice, berries, spinach, and ice and blend until the mixture is smooth and frothy. Serve in 4 glasses.

PER SERVING: 187 calories,
8 g fat (1 g saturated fat),
3 g protein, 27 mg sodium,
30 g carbohydrates, 19 g sugars
(0 g added sugar), 6 g fiber

VEGAN!

Creamy Strawberry & Orange Smoothie

Total time: 10 minutes
Makes: 1 serving

→ This dreamy smoothie is just what the doctor ordered! Metabolic syndrome, which affects up to one-third of all U.S. adults, is a cluster of conditions that together increase your risk for heart disease, stroke, and type 2 diabetes. A study at Oklahoma State University on obese adults with metabolic syndrome found that strawberries (the equivalent of three cups a day for eight weeks) could help lower total and LDL (bad) cholesterol.

INGREDIENTS
¾ cup orange juice, chilled
¼ cup whey protein powder
1 ¼ cups frozen strawberries
½ tablespoon honey
2 ice cubes

In a blender, combine orange juice, protein powder, strawberries, honey, and ice and blend until the mixture is smooth. Serve in a tall glass.

PER SERVING: 272 calories, 1 g fat (0 g saturated fat), 22 g protein, 46 mg sodium, 47 g carbohydrates, 33 g sugars (9 g added sugar), 5 g fiber

---

Health-Nut Smoothie

Total time: 10 minutes
Makes: 1 serving

→ We are nuts about this smoothie because it's so good-tasting and good for you! In addition to antioxidant-rich blueberries and omega-3-packed flaxseed, this elixir also has heart-healthy apples. Clinical trials have found that apples help lower LDL (bad) cholesterol and triglycerides. Be sure to keep the skin on the apple—it's where most of the fiber and flavonoids are.

INGREDIENTS
1 navel orange
½ cup plain low-fat yogurt
⅔ cup frozen blueberries
½ cup chopped apple
3 ice cubes
1 - 2 tablespoons ground flaxseed
Granola, for garnish

1. From orange, grate ½ teaspoon zest. Remove the remaining peel and white pith from orange and discard. Section orange.

2. In a blender, combine zest, orange sections, yogurt, blueberries, apple, ice, and flaxseed and blend until the mixture is smooth. Serve in a tall glass. Garnish with granola and enjoy.

PER SERVING: 318 calories, 7 g fat (2 g saturated fat), 11 g protein, 109 mg sodium, 58 g carbohydrates, 39 g sugars (1 g added sugar), 10 g fiber

BREAKFAST TO GO!

Great Grape Smoothie

Total time: 5 minutes
Makes: 1 serving

→ Here's an especially heart-healthy drink. Red grapes contain resveratrol, the same phytochemical found in red wine that protects against heart disease. The good news: The whole family can enjoy this delicious drink and reap the benefits!

INGREDIENTS
½ cup 100 percent red
    grape juice, chilled
¼ cup plain low-fat yogurt
1 cup frozen seedless red
    grapes

In a blender, combine grape juice, yogurt, and grapes and blend until the mixture is smooth. Serve in a tall glass.

PER SERVING: 223 calories,
1 g fat (0 g saturated fat),
4 g protein, 56 mg sodium,
52 g carbohydrates,
48 g sugars (0 g added sugar),
1 g fiber

Mighty Papaya Smoothie

Total time: 5 minutes
Makes: 1 serving

Tip **Whirl in a tablespoon of chia or hemp seeds for a hit of healthy fats.**

→ Papaya and a touch of honey perfectly complement the earthy flavor of kale. Kale is part of the cruciferous family of veggies (like broccoli and cauliflower), which are all rich in glucosinolates. This compound helps protect kale in nature, and lab studies have shown that glucosinolates also have a protective effect on our cells. Even more reason to throw some of the green stuff into your smoothie!

In a blender, combine papaya, kale, yogurt, oat milk, and honey and blend until the mixture is smooth. Serve in a tall glass.

PER SERVING: 296 calories, 9 g fat (4 g saturated fat), 14 g protein, 128 mg sodium, 44 g carbohydrates, 36 g sugar (9 g added sugar), 4 g fiber

INGREDIENTS

1 cup frozen papaya chunks
1 cup coarsely chopped kale, ribs removed
½ cup vanilla whole-milk Greek yogurt
½ cup unsweetened oat milk
½ teaspoon honey

Peachy-Cantaloupe Juice

Total time: 15 minutes
Makes: 5 servings

→ Sweet and fragrant, cantaloupe juice makes a delicious heart-smart drink. One cup of the melon provides 417 milligrams of potassium, which helps lower sodium levels and relaxes blood pressure. This is the perfect sipper to balance out saltier offerings (we're looking at you, bacon and lox!) at breakfast or brunch.

INGREDIENTS

1 large cantaloupe (2½ pounds), chilled
1 cup peach nectar or apricot nectar, chilled
1 tablespoon fresh lime juice
Lime slices, for garnish (optional)

1. Slice cantaloupe in half. Scoop out and discard the seeds. Remove the rind, then cut cantaloupe into 1-inch chunks.

2. In a blender, combine cantaloupe, peach or apricot nectar, and lime juice until smooth. Increase the speed to high; blend 1 minute. Pour into 5 glasses. Garnish with lime slices, if desired.

PER SERVING: 67 calories, 0 g fat (0 g saturated fat), 1 g protein, 22 mg sodium, 17 g carbohydrates, 15 g sugars (5 g added sugar), 1 g fiber

VEGAN & BRUNCH PICK!

Citrusy Gazpacho Sipper

Total time: 5 minutes, plus chilling time
Makes: 2 servings

→ The cold, tomato-based soup is the inspiration for this blender juice, which adds in a sweet note from freshly squeezed orange juice. With heart-protective lycopene in the tomato and plenty of potassium from the oranges and celery, you can feel great knowing that you're starting the day deliciously on a heart-smart note.

INGREDIENTS
2 large oranges
1 large ripe tomato, cored
    and quartered
2 large stalks celery, peeled
    and sliced
1 cup ice cubes

1. Squeeze juice from oranges into a blender. Add tomato, celery, and ice and blend until smooth.

2. Refrigerate until very cold, at least 1 hour. Serve in 2 tall glasses.

PER SERVING: 75 calories, 0.5 g fat (0 g saturated fat), 2 g protein, 57 mg sodium, 17 g carbohydrates, 12 g sugars (0 g added sugar), 2 g fiber

---

Celery Juice

VEGAN!

Total time: 5 minutes
Makes: 1 serving

→ Celery juice has been touted for doing everything from curing disease to causing dramatic weight loss. While those claims aren't true, celery juice still has a whole lot of green potential. First, celery contains a phytochemical called phthalides, which relaxes the tissues of artery walls, helping to increase blood flow and reduce blood pressure. And at 95 percent water, it's also incredibly hydrating!

INGREDIENTS
5 stalks celery
1 Granny Smith apple,
    cored and chopped
½ English cucumber
¾ cup coconut water,
    chilled

1. In a blender, combine celery, apple, cucumber, and coconut water.

2. Blend until the mixture is smooth. Strain and pour into a tall glass.

PER SERVING: 170 calories, 0 g fat (0 g saturated fat), 2 g protein, 175 mg sodium, 30 g carbohydrates, 25 g sugars (0 g added sugar), 4 g fiber

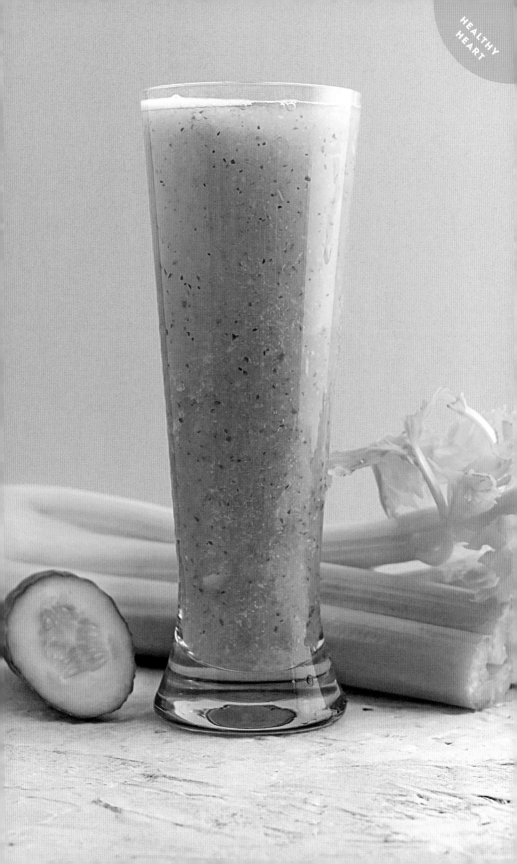

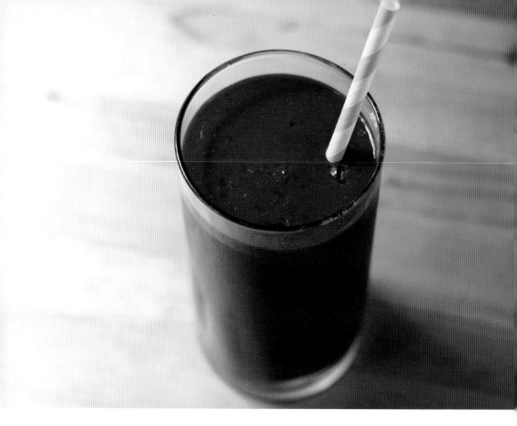

Beet Red Refresher

Total time: 10 minutes
Makes: 2 servings

➜ This scarlet juice is as delicious as it is gorgeous. And beets are chock-full of nutrients, including magnesium, which is key in keeping your heart healthy. The ruby-red root vegetable also aids in preventing heart disease with the plant pigment betalain, which has antioxidant and anti-inflammatory benefits.

INGREDIENTS

2 cups fresh strawberries (about 8 ounces), hulled and quartered

1 ½ cups cold water

1 cup sliced precooked beets (do not use canned)

½ small Granny Smith apple, peeled and thinly sliced

3 tablespoons fresh lemon juice

1 tablespoon agave nectar

In a blender, combine strawberries, water, beets, apple, lemon juice, and agave and blend until smooth. Serve in 2 tall glasses.

PER SERVING: 122 calories, 1 g fat (0 g saturated fat), 2 g protein, 67 mg sodium, 30 g carbohydrates, 24 g sugars (8 g added sugar), 4 g fiber

Tip **You can use maple syrup or honey in place of the agave nectar.**

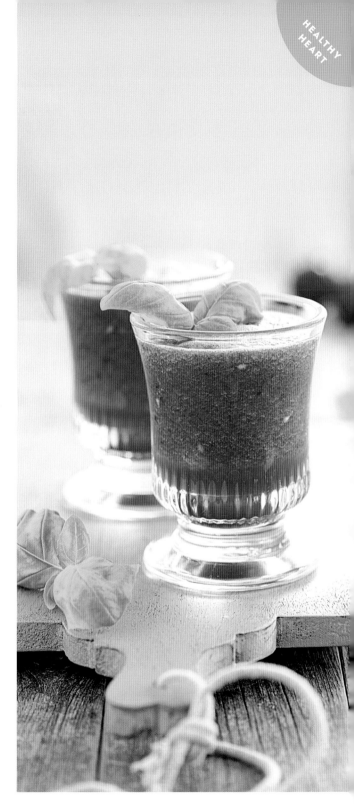

VEGAN!

Pink Basil Blend

Total time: 10 minutes
Makes: 2 servings

➜ This watermelon-based juice harnesses the flavor of summer, no matter what season it is. With its lycopene-rich melon and beta-carotene-packed carrots, you'll want to raise a glass of this sweet juice to heart health!

INGREDIENTS

3 cups watermelon chunks
1 cup freshly grated, peeled carrot
½ cup loosely packed fresh basil leaves, plus more for garnish
2 teaspoons fresh lemon juice
Pinch of salt

In a blender, combine watermelon, carrot, basil, lemon juice, and salt and blend until smooth. Pour into 2 tall glasses, garnish with basil, and serve.

PER SERVING: 85 calories, 0 g fat (0 g saturated fat), 2 g protein, 103 mg sodium, 26 g carbohydrates, 22 g sugars (0 g added sugar), 3 g fiber

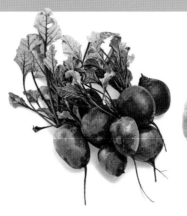
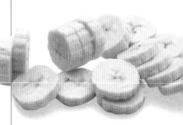

TOP 5 NUTRIENTS FOR HEART HEALTH

1. MAGNESIUM

New research points to magnesium as essential for keeping your heart healthy. Studies have shown a link between magnesium deficiency and high blood pressure. And people who don't get enough of this mineral have elevated inflammation markers in the body, which, as you know, can increase your risk for heart disease and other serious health conditions.

Women ages 31 and over need 320 milligrams per day (younger women require slightly less); men 31 and over plus (younger men need a bit less) require 420 milligrams.

Where to get it:

Beets, raw (1 cup): 31 mg

Almonds (1 ounce; 23 almonds): 77 mg

Spinach, cooked (1 cup): 157 mg

Banana (large): 37 mg

Avocado (half): 36 mg

2. POTASSIUM

We've mentioned potassium quite a bit in this chapter, so you already know how vital it is for heart health! Potassium helps balance out sodium levels in the body, contributing to a lower risk for heart disease. If you get your five to nine servings of fruits and veggies each day, it should be easy for you to knock out this requirement.

Women ages 19 and over need 2,600 milligrams per day; men require 3,400 milligrams.

Where to get it:

Banana (large): 487 mg

Potatoes (medium, with skin): 620 mg

Milk (8 ounces): 366 mg

Orange juice (8 ounces): 448 mg

Peach (large): 332 mg

Winter squash, cooked (1 cup): 582 mg

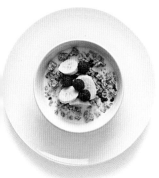

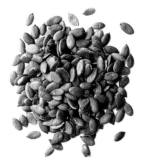

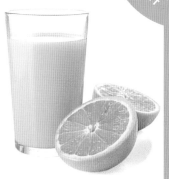

3. FOLIC ACID

The B vitamin folic acid is essential for heart health (and also for a healthy pregnancy). Folic acid regulates levels of homocysteine, a marker for heart disease, in the blood. Homocysteine damages blood vessel walls and can lead to blood clots.

Both women and men 19 and over need 400 micrograms per day.

Where to get it:
Fortified cereal (such as Total; 1 cup): 400 mcg

Lentils, cooked (1 cup): 358 mcg

Spinach, cooked (1 cup): 263 mcg

Edamame, cooked (1 cup): 200 mcg

Wheat germ (2 tablespoons): 85 mcg

4. NIACIN

Another B vitamin, niacin is beneficial for heart health because it helps to increase HDL (good) cholesterol levels.

Women ages 19 and over need 14 milligrams per day; men need 16 milligrams.

Where to get it:
Avocado (half): 1.75 mg

Peanut butter (2 tablespoons): 4.3 mg

Green peas (1 cup): 3 mg

Baked potato (large): 4.2 mg

Pumpkin seeds (1 ounce): 1.3 mg

5. CALCIUM

While we think of calcium as a bone-building mineral, it's also beneficial for heart health. Calcium, along with magnesium and potassium, helps regulate blood pressure. Calcium plays a role in weight management, too, which is also smart for your heart.

Women ages 19 to 50 need 1,000 milligrams per day, and women over 50 require 1,200 milligrams. Men 19 to 70 need 1,000 milligrams, and men over 70 require 1,200 milligrams.

Where to get it:
Milk (8 ounces): 300 mg

Yogurt (1 cup): 499 mg

Cottage cheese (1 cup): 200 mg

Almonds (1 ounce; 23 almonds): 76 mg

Fortified orange juice (8 ounces): 350 mg

Kale, cooked (2 cups): 359 mg

Chapter 5

Strong Muscles

Have you ever heard the saying that muscles are made in the kitchen? It sounds kind of silly at first. After all, unless you're putting in the time at the gym, in the studio, or at the park, you can't expect to gain muscle. But the truth is that without proper nutrition, all your sweat and effort won't lead to meaningful results.

The great thing is that with a little nutrition know-how, you can easily optimize your workouts and build strength. Pre- and post-workout smoothies are an amazing and delicious way to support your exercise routine. Properly fueling before and after a sweat session can make all the difference when it comes to creating success and feeling stronger. Get blending and get after it!

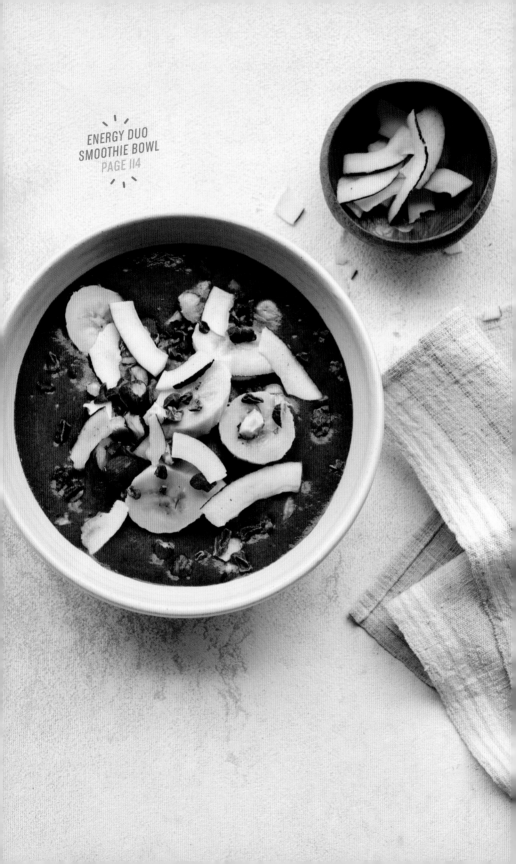

ENERGY DUO
SMOOTHIE BOWL
PAGE 114

Workout Recovery Smoothie

Total time: 10 minutes
Makes: 1 serving

➔ The ingredients in this cherry-vanilla smoothie can help you feel your best after a tough workout. Cherry juice has been shown to relieve post-exercise pain in athletes, while pomegranate juice can help accelerate muscle recovery. Beets are rich in nitrates, which some studies show can increase muscle function and lower blood pressure. A scoop of protein powder will help repair and build muscle tissue, and walnuts will keep your post-workout appetite under control.

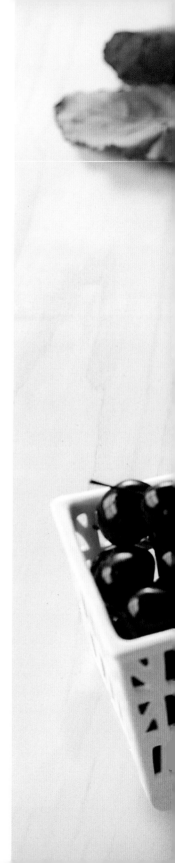

INGREDIENTS

¾ cup ice

¼ cup fresh or frozen pitted tart cherries

¼ cup pomegranate juice

1 scoop vanilla protein powder (turn to page 13 for a guide to picking the best one for you)

1 tablespoon chopped walnuts

1 small cooked, peeled beet (or raw beet, scrubbed and chopped)

In a blender, combine ice, cherries, pomegranate juice, protein powder, walnuts, and beet until smooth. Serve in a tall glass.

PER SERVING: 233 calories, 6 g fat (1.5 g saturated fat), 25 g protein, 107 mg sodium, 20 g carbohydrates, 16 g sugars (0 g added sugar), 2 g fiber

POST-WORKOUT SMOOTHIE CHECKLIST

☑ Protein to help repair microtears in muscles

☑ Carbohydrates to restore muscle glycogen reserves

☑ Antioxidants to fight oxidative damage caused by exercise

☑ Good fats to provide richness and satiety and to absorb fat-soluble vitamins

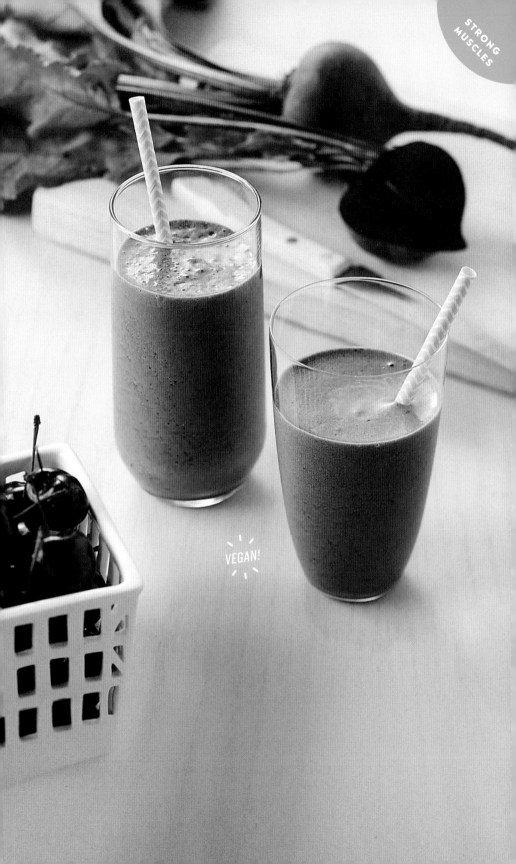

VEGAN!

Blueberry Cobbler Smoothie Bowl

Total time: 10 minutes
Makes: 2 servings

➜ Research shows that consuming protein immediately after a workout helps accelerate muscle growth and repair damaged muscle tissue. This tasty smoothie bowl delivers the right amount of protein to do just that.

VEGAN!

INGREDIENTS

FOR SMOOTHIE
1 cup frozen blueberries
½ cup unsweetened almond milk
1½ scoops protein powder
2 tablespoons almond butter
1 teaspoon vanilla extract

FOR TOPPING
½ cup fresh blueberries
¼ cup vanilla granola
2 tablespoons sliced almonds
2 teaspoons hemp seeds
1 teaspoon ground cinnamon

1. Combine blueberries, almond milk, protein powder, almond butter, and vanilla extract in a blender and blend until the mixture is smooth. Divide between 2 bowls.

2. Spoon ¼ cup blueberries onto each smoothie bowl. Top each with 2 tablespoons granola, 1 tablespoon almonds, and 1 teaspoon hemp seeds. Sprinkle with ½ teaspoon cinnamon and serve.

PER SERVING: 372 calories, 17 g fat (2.5 g saturated fat), 25 g protein, 132 mg sodium, 32 g carbohydrates, 16 g sugars (4 g added sugar), 7 g fiber

VEGAN!

Energy Duo Smoothie Bowl

Total time: 10 minutes
Makes: 2 servings

➡ Need some get-up-and-go before a workout? Reach for this smoothie about 15 minutes before exercise. It will take that long for the caffeine to kick in. And it doesn't just wake you up; caffeine increases dopamine, a neurotransmitter that enhances focus and lets you work out harder without feeling like it's a struggle. Bonus: The fiber—40 percent of your recommended daily intake (RDI)—stabilizes blood sugar to curb cravings. See photo, page 109.

FOR SMOOTHIE
1 cup coffee ice cubes
   (see below)
¾ cup unsweetened
   almond milk
¼ cup unsweetened cocoa
   powder
1 scoop protein powder
1 teaspoon vanilla extract
1 banana

FOR TOPPING
2 tablespoons cacao nibs
2 tablespoons hazelnuts,
   roughly chopped
2 tablespoons
   unsweetened coconut
½ banana, sliced

1. Blend ice cubes, almond milk, cocoa, protein powder, vanilla extract, and banana in a blender until the mixture is smooth. Divide between 2 bowls.

2. Sprinkle 1 tablespoon each cacao nibs, hazelnuts, and coconut onto each smoothie bowl. Top each with half the banana slices and serve.

PER SERVING: 347 calories, 18.5 g fat (8.5 g saturated fat), 18 g protein, 101 mg sodium, 34 g carbohydrates, 13 g sugars (0 g added sugar), 10 g fiber

> *Tip*
> It's easy to make coffee ice cubes, which are perfect for smoothies and for keeping iced coffee cold without diluting it. Simply brew a pot of coffee, then let it cool to room temperature. Pour the cooled coffee into an ice cube tray and place in the freezer. Once frozen, the ice cubes will last up to two weeks.

Potassium Peppermint Smoothie

Total time: 5 minutes, plus soaking time
Makes: 1 serving

→ Every tough workout deserves an equally great reward. Treat yourself with this minty smoothie, packed with muscle-building protein to help you repair, refuel, and re-energize.

INGREDIENTS

1 small frozen banana, sliced
1 cup plain organic soy milk
¼ cup fresh mint leaves
¼ cup raw cashews (soaked overnight)
⅓ cup silken tofu
¼ teaspoon vanilla extract
1 cup ice
Chopped cashews and/or rolled oats, for garnish (optional)

In a blender, combine banana, soy milk, mint leaves, cashews, tofu, vanilla extract, and ice until smooth. Top with a sprinkle of chopped cashews and/or rolled oats, if desired. Serve in a tall glass.

PER SERVING: 370 calories, 19 g fat (3 g saturated fat), 17 g protein, 78 mg sodium, 37 g carbohydrates, 15 g sugars (0 g added sugar), 12 g fiber

Tip
Soaking the cashews in advance helps them blend up nice and creamy. If you forgot to soak them overnight, don't fret! Simply place them in a microwave-safe container, cover with water, and microwave on high for 2 minutes. Drain and add the nuts to your smoothie.

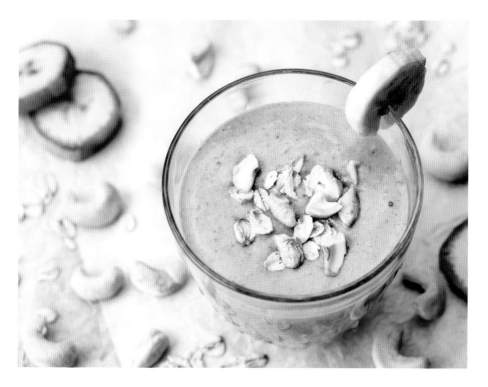

Strawberry-Avocado Refresher

Total time: 5 minutes
Makes: 1 serving

→ This creamy and delicious smoothie harnesses the nutrients in two superfoods: strawberries and avocados. One cup of the berries contains 110 percent of your vitamin C requirement for the day, and half of an avocado delivers 533 milligrams of potassium. Studies show that athletic performance is diminished when vitamin C levels are low. Potassium helps you maintain a healthy fluid balance and is essential for muscle contractions, as well as a healthy heart. Together, these two fruits make a super snack that's perfect for everyday athletes.

INGREDIENTS

1 cup halved strawberries
½ avocado, pitted and
    peeled
½ large frozen banana
Juice of half a lime
Handful of ice

Blend strawberries, avocado, banana, lime juice, and ice until smooth. Serve in a tall glass.

PER SERVING: 276 calories, 15.5 g fat (2 g saturated fat), 4 g protein, 10 mg sodium, 38 g carbohydrates, 17 g sugars (0 g added sugar), 12 g fiber

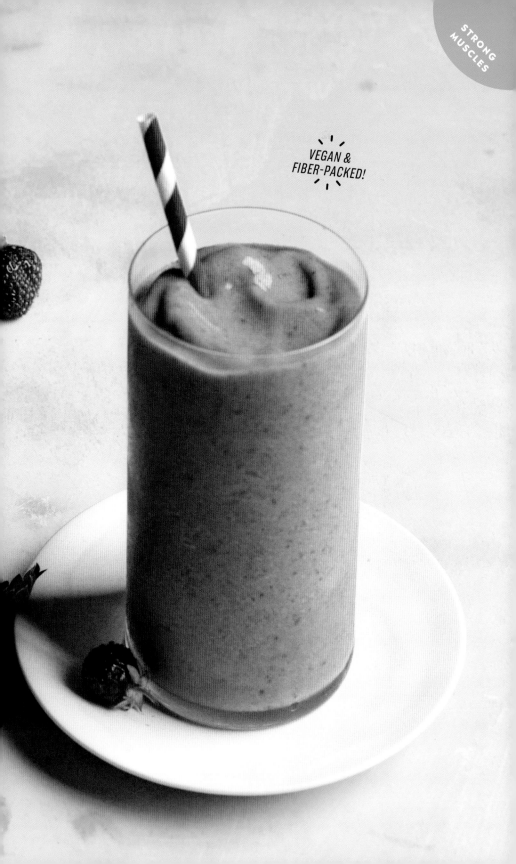

VEGAN &
FIBER-PACKED!

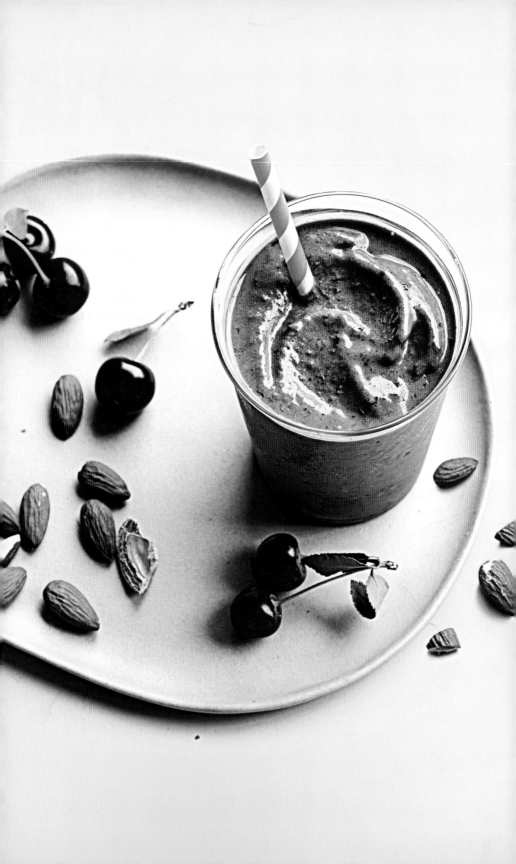

Cherry-Almond Smoothie

Total time: 5 minutes
Makes: 1 serving

➜ Drink up to get moving! This creamy, fruity blend contains ingredients that help ease joint and muscle pain. Tart cherry juice has been shown to minimize arthritis pain and post-exercise muscle soreness by reducing inflammation. Almond butter and yogurt contain magnesium, which helps relax tight muscles. And collagen powder contains amino acids to build bone and joint tissue and could help reduce osteoarthritis-related knee pain.

INGREDIENTS

1 cup 2 percent Greek yogurt
½ cup frozen Bing cherries
½ cup tart cherry juice
2 tablespoons almond butter
1-2 tablespoons collagen powder

In a blender, combine yogurt, cherries, cherry juice, almond butter, and collagen powder until smooth. Serve in a tall glass.

PER SERVING: 485 calories, 23 g fat (4 g saturated fat), 40 g protein, 122 mg sodium, 44 g carbohydrates, 32 g sugars (0 g added sugar), 5 g fiber

Tip
Collagen is a type of protein naturally found in our skin, tendons, cartilage, and connective tissue. Collagen also helps promote gut health. As we age, our bodies produce less of it, which can lead to sagging skin and also painful joints. You can find all types of collagen supplements made from beef, chicken, fish, and even eggshell membranes. Some are flavored and can be mixed with water, while others are plain and are better blended into a smoothie. We recommend looking for one that is sourced from grass-fed animals that haven't been treated with hormones.

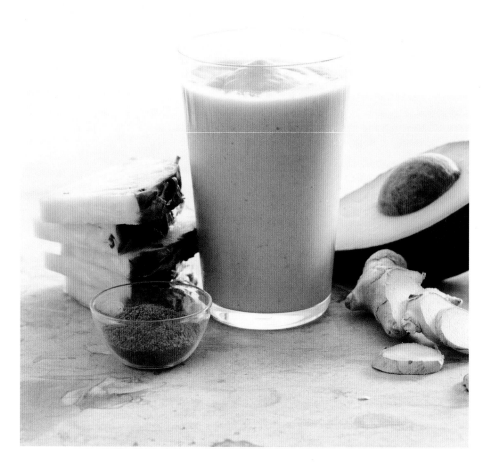

Sweet 'n' Spicy Tropical Smoothie

Total time: 10 minutes
Makes: 2 servings

→ Ginger has long been touted for its ability to help strengthen immunity. And it's also a powerful pain reducer. Combined with the electrolytes in coconut water, the spicy kick from cayenne, and the muscle-repairing benefits of whey protein, this post-workout smoothie will fix you up right!

INGREDIENTS
½ cup coconut water
2 tablespoons lemon juice
1 ripe avocado, pitted and peeled
1 scoop unsweetened whey protein powder
¼ teaspoon cayenne powder
2-inch piece fresh ginger, peeled and chopped
1 cup frozen pineapple and/or mango

In a blender, combine coconut water, lemon juice, avocado, protein powder, cayenne, ginger, and pineapple or mango. Serve in 2 tall glasses.

PER SERVING: 280 calories, 15.5 g fat (2.5 g saturated fat), 11 g protein, 91 mg sodium, 28 g carbohydrates, 14 g sugars (0 g added sugar), 9 g fiber

Green Apple Smoothie

Total time: 5 minutes
Makes: 1 serving

→ Runners have higher iron needs than the average person because they lose more of this vital mineral through wear and tear, sweat, and loss through the GI system. When you're low in iron, you can't make enough red blood cells, leading to less oxygen being transported to your muscles. Help replenish your stores with this protein- and iron-packed sipper.

INGREDIENTS

½ green apple, cored and chopped
1 cup baby spinach
1 scoop unsweetened whey protein powder
1 tablespoon nut butter
¾ cup water
Handful of ice (optional)

In a blender, combine apple, spinach, protein powder, nut butter, water, and ice (if using) until smooth. Serve in a tall glass.

PER SERVING: 230 calories, 10 g fat (2 g saturated fat), 21 g protein, 112 mg sodium, 20 g carbohydrates, 11 g sugars (0 g added sugar), 5 g fiber

PROTEIN-PACKED!

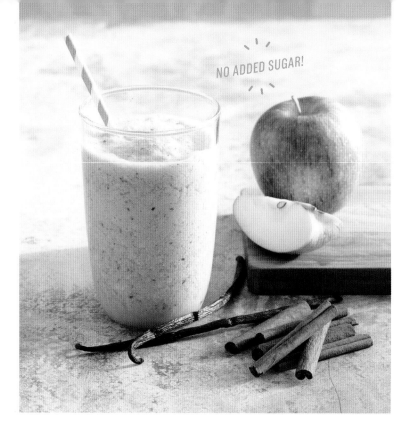

NO ADDED SUGAR!

Apple Spice Smoothie

Total time: 5 minutes
Makes: 2 servings

→ The online community is in love with apple cider vinegar (ACV), and it's become hugely popular with athletes. Lots of runners like taking a shot of ACV before a run because it's touted as a muscle cramp preventer and an inflammation fighter. While these benefits haven't been proven by science, there is evidence that ACV does help prevent spikes in blood glucose. And studies have found that cinnamon helps fight inflammation, making this an awesome pre- or post-run drink.

INGREDIENTS

¼ cup coconut water
1 tablespoon apple cider vinegar
1 teaspoon vanilla extract
½ cup plain Greek yogurt
½ teaspoon ground cinnamon
½ large apple, cored and chopped
¾ cup ice

In a blender, combine coconut water, apple cider vinegar, vanilla extract, yogurt, cinnamon, apple, and ice. Blend until smooth. Serve in 2 tall glasses.

PER SERVING: 93 calories, 2.5 g fat (1.5 g saturated fat), 5 g protein, 54 mg sodium, 13 g carbohydrates, 9 g sugars, (0 g added sugar), 2 g fiber

PROTEIN-PACKED!

Banana-Almond Protein Smoothie

Total time: 5 minutes
Makes: 2 servings

→ Post-workout is the most important time for muscle-building. If you don't replenish your body after a tough sweat session, you won't see the results from all your hard work. This yummy smoothie delivers 21 grams of protein to help repair microtears in your muscles and get them ready for your next run or spin.

INGREDIENTS

½ cup coconut water
½ cup plain Greek yogurt
3 tablespoons almond butter
1 scoop whey protein powder
1 tablespoon hulled hemp seeds
1 frozen banana
1 cup ice

In a blender, combine coconut water, yogurt, almond butter, protein powder, hemp seeds, banana, and ice. Serve in 2 tall glasses.

PER SERVING: 329 calories, 17 g fat (3 g saturated fat), 21 g protein, 159 mg sodium, 26 g carbohydrates, 15 g sugars (0 g added sugar), 5 g fiber

Café Mocha Smoothie

Total time: 5 minutes
Makes: 2 servings

➜ Dark winter mornings can make getting up for a workout challenging. But this shake will wake you up and keep you energized for hours.

INGREDIENTS

¾ cup chilled or cold-brewed coffee such as Perfect Cold-Brewed Coffee (see below)

3 tablespoons whole milk or milk of your choice

1 scoop unsweetened whey protein powder

1 tablespoon unsweetened cocoa powder

1 frozen banana, sliced

1 cup ice

In a blender, combine coffee, milk, protein powder, cocoa, banana, and ice and blend until the mixture is smooth. Serve in 2 tall glasses.

PER SERVING: 128 calories, 2 g fat (1 g saturated fat), 11 g protein, 36 mg sodium, 19 g carbohydrates, 10 g sugars (0 g added sugar), 2 g fiber

---

PERFECT COLD-BREWED COFFEE

Makes: ¾ cup

Cold brewing reduces the acidity of coffee, which in turn enhances its sweetness and other complex flavor notes. Feel free to double the ingredients if you'd like to have extra cold-brew on hand.

1. In a small pitcher or 1-quart measuring cup, whisk together ⅓ cup ground coffee and 1 ⅓ cups cold water until all lumps are gone.

2. Cover tightly and refrigerate for at least 5 hours, and ideally overnight (but not longer, or it will turn bitter).

3. Strain the coffee through a coffee-filter-lined strainer, pushing it through with a spatula.

4. Transfer cold brew to an airtight jar and store in the refrigerator for up to one week.

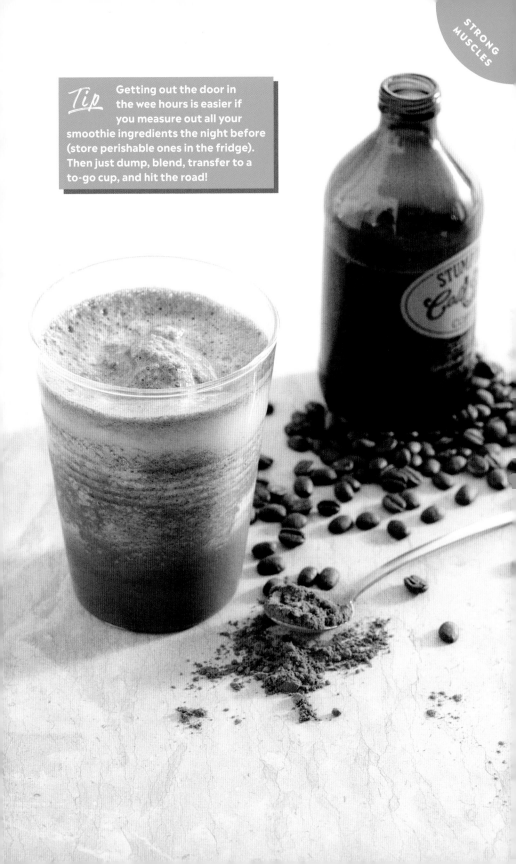

Tip Getting out the door in the wee hours is easier if you measure out all your smoothie ingredients the night before (store perishable ones in the fridge). Then just dump, blend, transfer to a to-go cup, and hit the road!

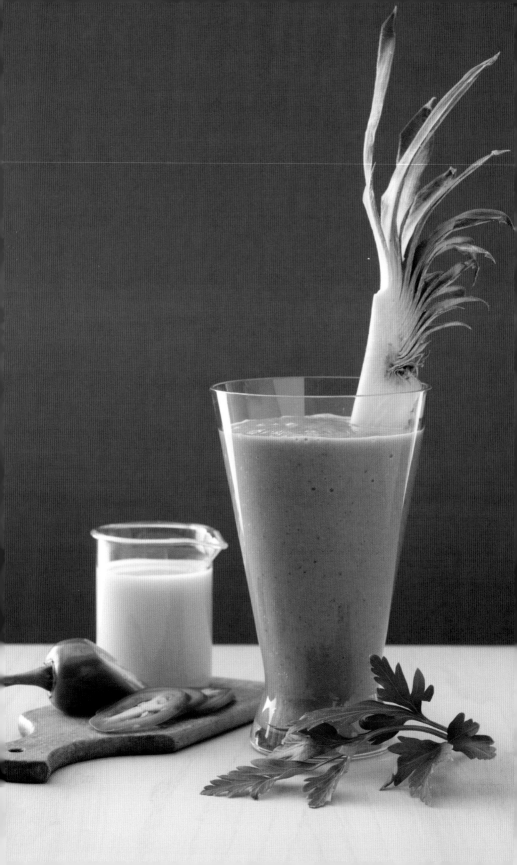

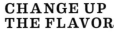

Banana-Avocado Zinger

Total time: 10 minutes
Makes: 2 servings

→ Need a pre-workout pick-me-up? Get revved naturally with B vitamins, which are plentiful in bananas, avocado, spinach, and parsley. Pineapple provides manganese, a mineral that's essential for energy production.

INGREDIENTS

½ cup chilled coconut water
1 chopped frozen banana
1 small avocado, pitted and peeled
½ cup baby spinach leaves
½ cup frozen pineapple chunks
¼ cup chopped fresh parsley
2 tablespoons fresh lime juice

In a blender, combine coconut water, banana, avocado, spinach, pineapple, parsley, and lime juice until smooth. Serve in 2 tall glasses.

PER SERVING: 217 calories, 11 g fat (2 g saturated fat), 3 g protein, 37 mg sodium, 31 g carbohydrates, 11 g sugars (0 g added sugar), 8 g fiber

CHANGE UP THE FLAVOR

The Banana-Avocado Zinger—or any of your favorite smoothie recipes—can be modified with these tasty ideas:

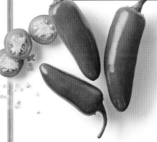

Kick the heat up a notch with metabolism-stoking minced fresh jalapeño. Start with a smidge of the pepper and adjust to taste.

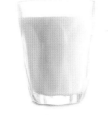

Substitute milk or a nondairy beverage for the coconut water, or blend in unsweetened whey protein powder to pump up the protein.

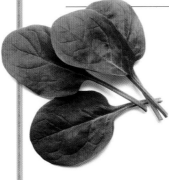

Throw in more spinach and/or parsley (or other leafy greens) for more iron.

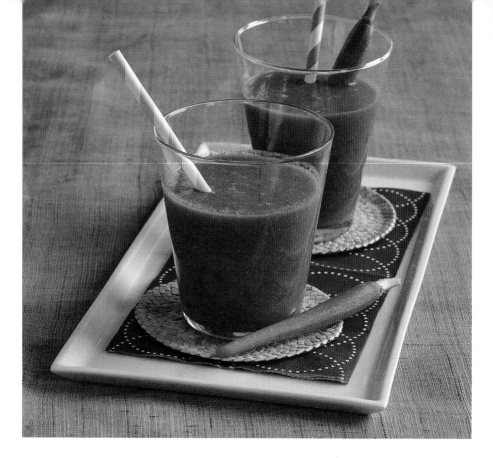

Tropical Twist Smoothie

Total time: 10 minutes
Makes: 2 servings

→ Coconut water is the slightly sweet liquid found in the center of a young, green coconut. It's a rich source of electrolytes, such as potassium, which help you rehydrate and prevent muscle cramping post-workout.

INGREDIENTS

1 cup pineapple chunks
¾ cup grated carrot
½ cup coconut water, chilled
½ cup ice cubes
2 tablespoons unsweetened dried coconut flakes, toasted
2 teaspoons agave nectar or honey
2 teaspoons white chia seeds
½ teaspoon ground turmeric (optional)

In a blender, combine pineapple, carrots, coconut water, ice, coconut flakes, agave or honey, chia seeds, and turmeric (if using) and blend until smooth. Pour into 2 glasses.

PER SERVING: 139 calories, 4.5 g fat (3 g saturated fat), 2 g protein, 47 mg sodium, 25 g carbohydrates, 18 g sugars (5 g added sugar), 4 g fiber

Tip Pineapple contains manganese, which is a trace mineral that's necessary for bone health. Manganese is a co-factor in the formation of bone cartilage and bone collagen, as well as bone mineralization.

Berry Satisfying Smoothie

Total time: 5 minutes
Makes: 2 servings

→ Add fiber-rich oats to a morning smoothie? Absolutely! They make it extra filling and provide whole-grain nutrients, plus slow-burning carbs to power you through your workout.

INGREDIENTS

2 cups frozen mixed berries
1 cup vanilla low-fat yogurt
1 ripe banana, sliced
½ cup quick-cooking oats
½ cup orange juice

In a blender, combine berries, yogurt, banana, oats, and orange juice and blend until the mixture is smooth. Serve in 2 glasses.

PER SERVING: 335 calories, 4 g fat (1 g saturated fat), 12 g protein, 82 mg sodium, 68 g carbohydrates, 41 g sugars (8 g added sugar), 8 g fiber

Tip You can either use quick-cooking oats or rolled oats (aka old-fashioned oats) in this recipe. Steel cut oats are too coarse to blend.

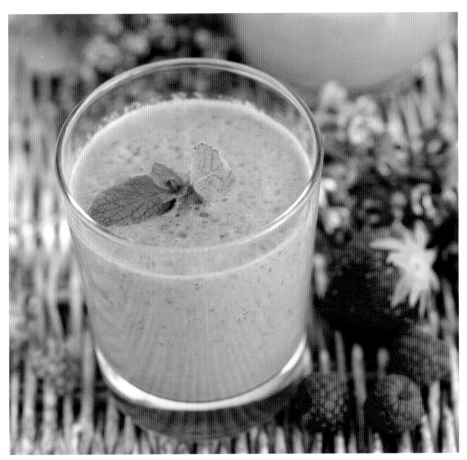

Strawberry-Chia Smoothie

Total time: 10 minutes
Makes: 1 serving

➜ OJ isn't the only way to get your vitamin C in the morning. Kiwis and strawberries are also good sources, and this fruity blend with chia seeds is custom-made to rev up your day. The chia seeds hold on to water, making this an especially hydrating post-workout drink.

INGREDIENTS
1 cup frozen strawberries
2 kiwifruits, peeled and chopped
¾ cup milk of your choice
1 tablespoon chia seeds
1 teaspoon ground ginger
4 ice cubes

In a blender, combine strawberries, kiwifruits, milk, chia seeds, ginger, and ice and blend until smooth. Serve in a tall glass.

PER SERVING: 305 calories, 10 g fat (4 g saturated fat), 10 g protein, 88 mg sodium, 48 g carbohydrates, 28 g sugars (0 g added sugar), 11 g fiber

Banana–Peanut Butter Smoothie

Total time: 10 minutes
Makes: 1 serving

➜ The classic childhood pairing of peanut butter and banana provides an awesome energy lift pre-workout.

INGREDIENTS
1 small ripe banana, cut in half
½ cup low-fat (1 percent) milk
1 teaspoon creamy peanut butter
1 teaspoon honey (optional)
3 ice cubes

In a blender, combine banana, milk, peanut butter, honey (if using), and ice and blend until the mixture is smooth. Serve in a tall glass.

PER SERVING: 173 calories, 4 g fat (1.5 g saturated fat), 6 g protein, 77 mg sodium, 30 g carbohydrates, 19 g sugars (0 g added sugar), 3 g fiber

Tip Stuck with a bunch of unripe bananas? Plan ahead and flash-ripen them in the freezer! The skin will turn black and the fruit will be fully ripe in a few hours. (Your smoothies will be colder and thicker too.) For more tips on ripening bananas, turn to page 22.

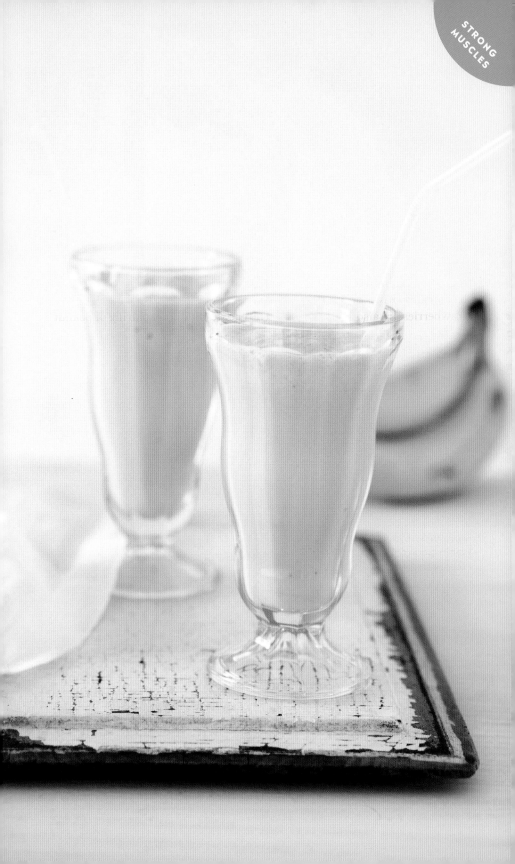

Tip This recipe is equally delish with cashew or walnut butter. And a dash of cinnamon would add another pop of antioxidants.

Java Blast Smoothie

Total time: 5 minutes
Makes: 1 serving

→ Trying to fit a HIIT workout into your hectic morning? This blender breakfast gives you a nice burst of nutrients while energizing you with a balance of protein, carbs, fiber, and healthy fats. Cocoa powder provides a dose of flavanols, which promote healthy circulation—a must for anyone who likes to be active.

INGREDIENTS

1 ripe banana, sliced
1 cup ice cubes
½ cup vanilla fat-free Greek yogurt
¼ cup Perfect Cold-Brewed Coffee (page 124)
1 teaspoon almond butter
2 teaspoons unsweetened cocoa powder
½ teaspoon vanilla extract

In a blender, combine banana, ice, yogurt, coffee, almond butter, cocoa powder, and vanilla extract and blend until the mixture is smooth. Serve in a tall glass.

PER SERVING: 248 calories, 4 g fat (1 g saturated fat), 14 g protein, 45 mg sodium, 43 g carbohydrates, 27 g sugars (7 g added sugar), 6 g fiber

Rise & Shine Smoothie

Total time: 5 minutes
Makes: 4 servings

→ Hot, humid weather calls for the most hydrating of smoothies. Wake up and whip up this golden smoothie packed with vitamins, minerals, protein, and healthy fats. Wheat germ adds a craveable nuttiness to this sipper, and the omega-3 fatty acids help lower inflammation, which is essential for athletes.

INGREDIENTS

1 large ripe banana
2 cups frozen pineapple chunks
2 cups ice cubes
1 cup orange juice
½ cup vanilla low-fat yogurt
¼ cup wheat germ

In a blender, combine banana, pineapple, ice, orange juice, yogurt, and wheat germ and blend until the mixture is smooth and frothy. Serve in 4 tall glasses.

PER SERVING: 158 calories, 1 g fat (0 g saturated fat), 5 g protein, 21 mg sodium, 34 g carbohydrates, 16 g sugars (2 g added sugar), 3 g fiber

Tip
Yes, you can eat ice pops for breakfast! Make a second batch of this zesty smoothie and pour it into ice-pop molds. Freeze for five to six hours or overnight. To unmold, run the pops briefly under warm water and remove.

Protein Power Smoothie

Total time: 5 minutes
Makes: 1 serving

➜ Blend up this fruity smoothie post-workout to deliver serious protein to your body. The whey protein and milk add up to a whopping 25 grams of protein, which is the perfect amount for your body to absorb at one time. Optimize muscle repair by sipping this within 15 minutes to 1 hour after your sweat session.

INGREDIENTS
¾ cup fat-free milk
½ ripe banana
½ cup frozen raspberries
½ cup frozen blueberries
1 scoop vanilla whey
      protein powder
5 ice cubes

In a blender, combine milk, banana, raspberries, blueberries, protein powder, and ice and blend until the mixture is smooth. Serve in a tall glass.

PER SERVING: 284 calories,
2 g fat (1 g saturated fat),
27 g protein, 148 mg sodium,
42 g carbohydrates,
26 g sugars (0 g added sugar),
7 g fiber

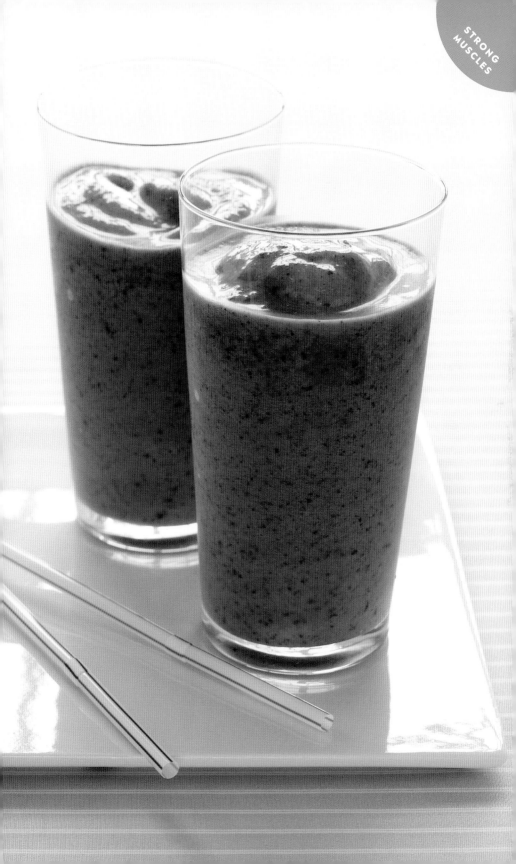

Cool as a Cucumber Smoothie

Total time: 5 minutes
Makes: 1 serving

➜ At 96 percent water, cucumber is one of the most hydrating ingredients you can find. Combine it with spinach, celery, banana, pineapple, and Greek yogurt for a super body boost post-workout.

INGREDIENTS

1 cup baby spinach
½ cup chopped cucumber
1 stalk celery, chopped
½ ripe banana, sliced
½ cup pineapple chunks
1 5.3-ounce container plain
    fat-free Greek yogurt
½ cup coconut water
4 ice cubes
Parsley for garnish, optional

In a blender, combine spinach, cucumber, celery, banana, pineapple, yogurt, coconut water, and ice and blend until the mixture is smooth. Serve in a tall glass, garnish with parsley, if using, and serve.

PER SERVING: 232 calories,
1 g fat (0 g saturated fat),
19 g protein, 164 mg sodium,
40 g carbohydrates, 26 g sugars
(0 g added sugar), 5 g fiber

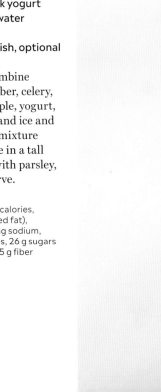

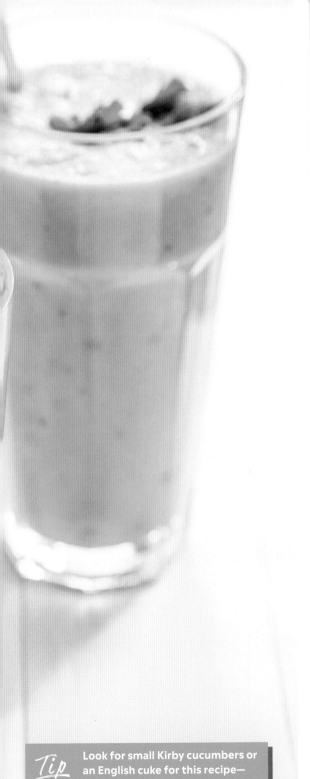

VEGAN!

Breakfast Jump Start

Total time: 5 minutes
Makes: 1 serving

→ It's smart to go simple before a morning workout—too much fiber can leave you running for the bathroom instead of running around the park. This smoothie will get you going without making you feel too full. And with nearly 30 percent of the potassium you need for the day, it's a sweet treat for your muscles too.

INGREDIENTS

1 cup almond or oat milk
1 frozen banana, sliced
1 cup strawberries, hulled
2 tablespoons wheat germ

In a blender, combine almond or oat milk, banana, strawberries, and wheat germ. Blend until the mixture is smooth. Serve in a tall glass.

PER SERVING: 248 calories, 5 g fat (1 g saturated fat), 7 g protein, 183 mg sodium, 48 g carbohydrates, 23 g sugars (0 g added sugar), 9 g fiber

Tip **Look for small Kirby cucumbers or an English cuke for this recipe—both are seedless.**

Cherry Vanilla Smoothie

Total time: 5 minutes
Makes: 2 servings

➜ Do you fit your workouts in at night? Evening sweat sessions might be cutting into your slumber. The science is inconclusive regarding whether exercising in the evening can disrupt your sleep cycle, but if you find yourself too wired after p.m. runs, sip on this smoothie before bed. Tart cherry juice is a potent source of melatonin, which helps ease you into a restful slumber—no pills required.

INGREDIENTS

¾ cup Montmorency (tart) cherry juice
1 cup vanilla non-fat Greek yogurt
1 cup ice
1 banana

In a blender, combine cherry juice, banana, yogurt, and ice. Blend until the mixture is smooth. Serve in 2 tall glasses.

PER SERVING: 129 calories, 0 g fat (0 g saturated fat), 11 g protein, 54 mg sodium, 21 g carbohydrates, 18 g sugars (6 g added sugar), 0 g fiber

HYDRATION 101

Staying hydrated is incredibly important when you're active. It allows your body to cool itself down without increasing your heart rate. The key to good hydration is a combination of water, electrolytes, and hydrating foods.

WATER:

If you're active on most days, aim to drink 3 liters (12½ cups) daily. Always bring a full water bottle with you on runs and walks and to fitness classes.

ELECTROLYTES:

You don't need to have a sports drink or an electrolyte mix unless you're exercising for more than an hour or sweating profusely. Your next meal or snack (like the Cool as a Cucumber Smoothie on page 136) should have enough sodium to replace what you've lost through sweat. You can always add a dash of sea salt to any smoothie if you're feeling depleted.

HYDRATING FOODS:

Water isn't the only way to hydrate! Most fruits and vegetables contain at least 80 percent water. Feel free to replace a few glasses of water with produce that's high in water content, or simply find smoothie recipes in this book with those ingredients. Here are the top produce picks:

CUCUMBER 96%
ICEBERG LETTUCE 96%
CELERY 95%
RADISH 95%
ZUCCHINI 95%
TOMATO 94%
STRAWBERRY 92%
WATERMELON 92%
GRAPEFRUIT 91%
CANTALOUPE 90%

INDEX

Note: Page numbers in *italics* indicate photos separate from recipes.

PHOTO CREDITS

HEARST
HOME

The information in this book is not meant to take the place of the advice of your doctor. Before embarking on a weight loss program, you are advised to seek your doctor's counsel to make sure that the weight loss plan you choose is right for your particular needs.

Cover design by Made Visible Studio
Book design by Made Visible Studio

Library of Congress Cataloging-in-Publication Data is available.

10 9 8 7 6 5 4 3 2 1

Published by Hearst Home, an imprint of Hearst Books/Hearst Magazine Media, Inc.
300 West 57th Street
New York, NY 10019

Prevention, Hearst Home, the Hearst Home logo, and Hearst Books are registered trademarks of Hearst Magazine Media, Inc.
Prevention is a registered trademark of Hearst Magazine, Inc.

For information about custom editions, special sales, premium and corporate purchases, please go to hearst.com/magazines/hearst-books

Printed in China
ISBN 978-1-950785-02-5